Lightning Injuries:
Electrical, Medical, and Legal Aspects

Editors

**Christopher J. Andrews, B.E.(Hons),
M.Eng.Sc., Dip.Comp.Sc., M.B.B.S.(Hons),
M.A.C.S., S.M.I.R.E.E., S.M.I.E.E.E.**
formerly Lecturer and Research Fellow
Department of Electrical Engineering
University of Queensland
St. Lucia, Australia
currently House Medical Officer
The Wesley Hospital
Brisbane, Australia
and medical practitioner in private practice

Mary Ann Cooper, M.D., F.A.C.E.P.
Associate Professor and Residency Research Director
Program in Emergency Medicine
University of Illinois Hospital
Chicago, Illinois

**Mat Darveniza, F.T.S., B.E., Ph.D.,
D.Eng., F.I.E.Aust., F.I.E.E.E.**
Professor in Electrical Engineering (Personal Chair)
Department of Electrical Engineering
University of Queensland
St. Lucia, Australia

David Mackerras, Ph.D.
Honorary Research Consultant
Department of Electrical Engineering
University of Queensland
St. Lucia, Australia

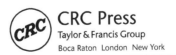

CRC Press
Taylor & Francis Group
Boca Raton London New York

CRC Press is an imprint of the
Taylor & Francis Group, an **informa** business

First published 1992 by CRC Press
Taylor & Francis Group
6000 Broken Sound Parkway NW, Suite 300
Boca Raton, FL 33487-2742

First issued in paperback 2020

Reissued 2018 by CRC Press

Library of Congress Cataloging-in-Publication Data

Lightning injuries / edited by Christopher J. Andrews . . . [et al.].
        p.   cm.
    Includes bibliographical references and index.
    ISBN 0-8493-5458-7
    1. Electricity, Injuries from. 2. Lightning — Health aspects.
    I. Andrews, Christopher J.
    RD96.5.L54   1992
    6 17.1'224—dc20

                                                                                91-35184

A Library of Congress record exists under LC control number: 91035184

Publisher's Note
The publisher has gone to great lengths to ensure the quality of this reprint but points out that some imperfections in the original copies may be apparent.

Disclaimer
The publisher has made every effort to trace copyright holders and welcomes correspondence from those they have been unable to contact.

ISBN 13: 978-0-367-57259-4 (pbk)
ISBN 13: 978-1-315-89494-2 (hbk)

Visit the Taylor & Francis Web site at http://www.taylorandfrancis.com and the
CRC Press Web site at http://www.crcpress.com

First published 1992 by CRC Press
Taylor & Francis Group
6000 Broken Sound Parkway NW, Suite 300
Boca Raton, FL 33487-2742

First issued in paperback 2020

Reissued 2018 by CRC Press

Library of Congress Cataloging-in-Publication Data

Lightning injuries / edited by Christopher J. Andrews . . . [et al.].
     p. cm.
    Includes bibliographical references and index.
    ISBN 0-8493-5458-7
    1. Electricity, Injuries from. 2. Lightning — Health aspects.
  I. Andrews, Christopher J.
  RD96.5.L54   1992
  6 17.1'224—dc20   91-35184

A Library of Congress record exists under LC control number: 91035184

ISBN 13: 978-0-367-57259-4 (pbk)
ISBN 13: 978-1-315-89494-2 (hbk)

Visit the Taylor & Francis Web site at http://www.taylorandfrancis.com and the
CRC Press Web site at http://www.crcpress.com

Lightning Injuries:
Electrical, Medical, and Legal Aspects

Editors

Christopher J. Andrews, B.E.(Hons),
M.Eng.Sc., Dip.Comp.Sc., M.B.B.S.(Hons),
M.A.C.S., S.M.I.R.E.E., S.M.I.E.E.E.
formerly Lecturer and Research Fellow
Department of Electrical Engineering
University of Queensland
St. Lucia, Australia
currently House Medical Officer
The Wesley Hospital
Brisbane, Australia
and medical practitioner in private practice

Mary Ann Cooper, M.D., F.A.C.E.P.
Associate Professor and Residency Research Director
Program in Emergency Medicine
University of Illinois Hospital
Chicago, Illinois

Mat Darveniza, F.T.S., B.E., Ph.D.,
D.Eng., F.I.E.Aust., F.I.E.E.E.
Professor in Electrical Engineering (Personal Chair)
Department of Electrical Engineering
University of Queensland
St. Lucia, Australia

David Mackerras, Ph.D.
Honorary Research Consultant
Department of Electrical Engineering
University of Queensland
St. Lucia, Australia

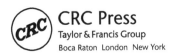

CRC Press
Taylor & Francis Group
Boca Raton London New York

CRC Press is an imprint of the
Taylor & Francis Group, an **informa** business

FOREWORD

While I greatly appreciate the opportunity of writing a foreword to *Lightning Injuries: Electrical, Medical, and Legal Aspects,* I should point out that my knowledge of lightning phenomena is associated with the physical rather than the medical side of the subject. Further, this knowledge was largely gained from the 1950s to the 1970s. A study of lightning fatalities in Australia toward the end of this period was relevant to the preparation of an Australian Manual on Lightning Protection, which included a section on personal safety during times of lightning activity. It is appropriate that this topic is fully dealt with in the present volume.

It is also fitting to remind readers that it is just 200 years since Benjamin Franklin died, and to recall his invention of the lightning rod and the innumerable lives it saved. Remarkably, his concept has probably undergone fewer subsequent changes than any other technical innovation of his period.

The editors are to be congratulated on attracting an exceptionally wide range of specialist contributors, thus providing a compendium of the latest information on the medical aspects of lightning injury — an area with many ramifications and uncertainties. The latter include the lack of means of estimating the strength of a lightning flash to ground as it affects a human being. In contrast, it is technically feasible, with special instrumentation, to obtain data on the magnitude of the current in a lightning flash to an inanimate object.

To achieve such a comprehensive coverage as the book provides, Dr. Andrews has clearly drawn on his experience both as an electrical engineer and as a medical practitioner. The outcome is that a balance has been struck between reporting the behavior of lightning as perceived by scientists and engineers and an analysis of its effect on the human body. In the latter connection, I am reminded of a statement by Dalziel in 1961 that, in spite of extensive research, the mechanism of death by lightning remains "entirely speculative". In 1976, Golde and Lee concluded that "while our knowledge of the physiological effects of lightning is not complete, the mechanisms by which it may cause death are fairly well understood…". Now, 15 years later, the most recent progress is well presented in this volume.

Emeritus Professor S. A. Prentice

PREFACE

This book sprang from a germ of an idea in early 1987 — an idea which was, in fact, initially quite different from the final form and content this published volume has grown to embody.

I had just been reemployed in the Academic Department of Electrical Engineering at the University of Queensland after an absence of several years. During that time, I had studied and practiced medicine, and in order to make use of both disciplines in which I had trained, was developing an interest in electromedicine. In a circuitous way, too long to relate here, my interest in lightning injuries was stirred and the fascination with these injuries began to grow.

At the same time, things at the University were changing. New building was occurring, and this entailed first the demolition of an old building inhabited by the Department since World War II. Much archival material was stored in the building and it was fascination itself to sift through it prior to the demolition. My former colleague, David Mackerras, had accumulated much material in his usual thorough way, but for me the material originating with Professor Sidney Prentice held particular interest.

While Professor Prentice taught me in the early 1970s, many others have great cause for gratitude to him. Many Queensland lightning researchers (all?) owe their beginnings and early training to him. It therefore gives me a great deal of satisfaction that he has agreed to write the foreword to this volume.

But Prentice's interests were not only in the physical aspects of lightning. He was among the first to publish a comprehensive examination of death and injury statistics. Remembering this, and my burgeoning interest in the medical aspects of lightning studies, I sought him out in his retirement. I spent an enjoyable morning sitting with him on his home veranda in Brisbane on a sunny tropical day being shown pieces of an amazing collection of accumulated material (from inevitable brown boxes!). Subsequently, it was Prentice who encouraged me to venture onto the international stage in my chosen area of interest, by presenting me with a brochure describing the 1988 Oklahoma Conference on Lightning and Static Electricity organized by Dr. Don McGorman. He also offered a curt, "You should go. And you should present" — both of which I did, with some trepidation and only because of his initiative.

Against this background, then, grew the original idea. Surely someone should bring together the wealth of material accumulated by Prentice and the Queensland group — a sort of collected works. But from there, the idea became bigger than its creator, and drove itself in a different direction.

I became very aware of the uniqueness of lightning injury, and the fact that this was not widely appreciated. Mary Ann Cooper was to play a significant role later in reinforcing this conception. The extant literature was patchy and ill synthesized. Misunderstandings abounded, and speculation was often wild. The most recent review of any comprehensiveness and quality was that of Mary Ann (her chapter in *Management of Wilderness and Environmental Emergencies* edited by Paul Auerbach et al.). The only book I had seen on the topic was Spencer's delightful but largely historic work from the 1930s. Here was a gap desperately needing to be filled. And so the idea progressed. Obvious among the Queensland group to contribute to the work were Mat Darveniza and David Mackerras. Their work needs no introduction and it has been my pleasure and good fortune to work with them — not only on this project. It was also a delight when Mary Ann (who no doubt several years ago wondered who on earth this brash young Australian pestering her with mail really was) joined the team, complementing the technical aspects of the work with her wide medical experience, perhaps the widest currently in the world. And so the editorial group was formed. I then set about harassing a group of experts, worldwide, asking them to contribute sections to the work from the perspective of their own special areas. The quality of the work has been immeasurably enhanced by their contributions, representing those of fine and noted scientists and clinicians in their fields.

I record my thanks to my long-suffering co-editors, and also to the patience of the many contributors over the last 2 years. They can be justly proud of the result. It is also a great pleasure to acknowledge the sympathetic and skillful guidance of Janice Morey and her staff at CRC.

What has been attempted here? The problem with research such as ours is that it spans two quite separate disciplines, different in content and language, and also in fundamental approach — the detailed analysis and modeling of the physical scientist contrasted with the often empirical approach, but also urgent need to treat an immediate problem of the clinical scientist. To find a common language in order to appreciate the respective approaches and contributions is only the first part of the problem. Without input from both sides of the fence, the understanding of and rational basis for therapy for lightning injury is diminished. Mary Ann has reinforced my own thinking along these lines and has been a welcome conscience for technocrats who might otherwise have "gone wild" in trying to communicate their perspective of the topic.

So in this volume we are attempting to bridge a gap. How successful we are remains to be seen, and feedback on this matter will be welcomed. The physical basis of lightning phenomena has been set out with a view to assisting the clinician in understanding the "hard" science underlying the problem. The symptomatology is set out, and an attempt has been made to synthesize the underlying pathophysiology of the injuries. In a sense, the writers of these latter sections have had the most difficult job. Little real pathophysiology is known with certainty, and speculation is rife. The contributors have had the difficult task of presenting what is known, synthesizing competing theories of what is speculative and adding their own critical appraisal, and then pointing to areas for fruitful research regarding what is not known. Treatment has been recommended based on current experience. Technologists will, it is hoped, benefit from the clinical sections, just as the clinicians will from the physical. Legal aspects are assuming greater importance, especially with regard to injuries thought to be transmitted via agencies under control of public utilities, and a chapter explores this matter. Telephone-mediated injury is a special interest of three of the editors and provides an archetype of the latter injury mechanism, and is thus included as an appendix.

The task has been a difficult and challenging one, and it is hoped that we have succeeded.

C. J. Andrews
Brisbane, Australia
December, 1990

EDITORS

Dr. Christopher John Andrews (Chris) was born in Tamworth, New South Wales, Australia, and was educated in Wagga Wagga, NSW, and Brisbane, Queensland. He attended Brisbane State High School and the University of Queensland.

In 1973, he graduated B.E. with first class honors in electrical engineering, and in 1976 was awarded the Master of Engineering Science degree by research, and the postgraduate Diploma of Computer Science. For 2 years he was employed as Senior Tutor in Computer Science, teaching at all levels and pursuing research interests in digital design and microprocessor interfacing.

In 1977, he returned to undergraduate study and was awarded the degrees M.B., B.S., with honors in 1982. He practiced medicine for 2 years full time, and then returned to the University of Queensland where he was employed as a research fellow and lecturer in electrical engineering. During this time, he developed a research interest in lightning and lightning injuries, first examining injuries to patients receiving a shock via the public telephone system. Wider aspects of lightning injury were subsequently added to the research program. Due to his interests in this area, he has become known as an international expert in medical aspects of lightning injury. He has published in the field, and also presented at international symposia in the area. He has also received international invitations to lecture on the subject. He has just submitted his Ph.D. thesis on lightning injuries.

In parallel with the university position, he also pursued part-time medical practice in intensive care medicine, returning full time to this practice in 1989. Currently, he continues the intensive care aspect of his practice and is in private medical practice otherwise. As part of this practice, he regularly is called on to assess and treat lightning-injured patients.

Chris is a senior member of IEEE and IREE, and a member of the Australian Computer Society (ACS).

He is married, with two sons aged five and two. Outside interests include the board of the children's kindergarten, photography, amateur radio, personal computing, fine music, and amateur theater.

Mary Ann Cooper, a native of Indiana, graduated magna cum laude from Michigan State University with a B.S. in biochemistry, and went on to receive her M.D. from the same university in 1974. She was ranked in the top 1% of her undergraduate class and was a member of Phi Beta Kappa. Since completing her years of education, she has garnered a number of awards, two of them for outstanding service in the area of emergency medicine. She has also been written up in *Who's Who of American Women*.

Dr. Cooper has directed, worked in, and trained others for a wide array of emergency medical services. She has been director of paramedics programs in Omaha, Nebraska, Louisville, Kentucky, and Hartford, Connecticut, and has taught emergency medicine at the University of Louisville and the University of Connecticut. She is currently an Associate Professor and Residency Research Director in the Program in Emergency Medicine at the University of Illinois in Chicago.

Through her extensive public service and professional involvements, Dr. Cooper has gained experience in many aspects of medical practice, including neonatal and pediatric intensive care, disaster preparedness, trauma care in the field and in the emergency room, and treatment of burns and electrical injuries.

She has written numerous articles on a variety of medical emergency topics, most notably on the care of lightning injuries, and has authored three books on related subjects. Dr. Cooper is an acknowledged authority on lightning injuries, and has appeared on local and national television and at dozens of lectures and conferences to discuss both the treatment of these injuries in particular and critical care in general.

Recently she has added a new responsibility to the many she already juggles: the care and treatment of her new baby.

Mat Darveniza, born in 1932 at Innisfail, Australia, is a graduate of the Universities of Queensland (B.E., 1953; D. Eng., 1980) London (Ph.D., 1959), and Chalmers University (Hon. D.Sc. Eng., 1990). He has worked in the electricity supply and manufacturing industries and at universities in Australia, U.S., Germany, Argentina, England, and Sweden.

Since joining the University of Queensland in 1959, his research and consulting interests have included lightning protection, high voltage and insulation engineering, and engineering education. He has over one hundred scientific and engineering publications, including a book entitled *The Electrical Properties of Wood and Line Design.* He is a regular contributor to international conferences and continuing education courses, often as the guest lecturer.

Professor Darveniza has a Personal Chair and between 1983 and 1987 was Head of the Department of Electrical Engineering. He is a Director of UniQuest Pty Ltd. and of NATA (National Association of Testing Authorities), Australia.

Professor Darveniza is a Fellow of IEEE, the IEAust, and the Australian Academy of Technological Sciences and Engineering.

He is married with three children. His recreations include music, squash/tennis, and surfing/ windsurfing.

David Mackerras was born in 1926 in Sydney, Australia, and is a graduate of the University of Sydney (B.Sc., 1950; Dip. Ed., 1952) and of Queensland (B.E. Honors, 1960; Ph.D., 1971). He has worked in the NSW Department of Education, in the electricity supply industry, and in the Electrical Engineering Department, University of Queensland (1961 to 1988).

Since joining the University of Queensland, his research interests have included a study of the occurrence and characteristics of lightning in southeast Queensland, lightning effects in telecommunication systems, and the analysis and display of speech characteristics for therapeutic and diagnostic purposes.

He has authored about 60 scientific and engineering publications and reports, mainly related to the above topics. He has carried out several major consultations relating to lightning damage prevention and protection from electromagnetic hazards for Telecom Australia, the Department of Defense, and other organizations.

Since retiring from the Electrical Engineering Department in December 1988, he has continued to serve on the Committee on Lightning Protection of the Standards Association of Australia, is continuing consulting work on lightning protection, and is continuing a joint project with Mat Darveniza on the worldwide survey of the cloud-flash-to-ground-flash ratio using CGR3 instruments.

CONTRIBUTORS

Christopher J. Andrews, B.E.(Hons), M.Eng.Sc., Dip.Comp.Sc., M.B.B.S.(Hons), M.A.C.S., S.M.I.R.E.E., S.M.I.E.E.E.
formerly Lecturer and Research Fellow
Department of Electrical Engineering
University of Queensland
St. Lucia, Australia
currently House Medical Officer
The Wesley Hospital
Brisbane, Australia
and medical practitioner *in private practice*

LaV. Bergstrom, M.D.
Professor of Surgery
Division of Head and Neck Surgery
Department of Surgery
University of California, Los Angeles

R. Cash, M.D.
Psychiatrist
Child and Family Therapy Unit
Royal Childrens Hospital
Brisbane, Australia

Mary Ann Cooper, M.D., F.A.C.E.P.
Associate Professor and Residency
  Research Director
Program in Emergency Medicine
University of Illinois Hospital
Chicago, Illinois

Mat Darveniza, F.T.S., B.E., Ph.D., D.Eng., F.I.E.Aust., F.I.E.E.E.
Professor in Electrical Engineering
  (Personal Chair)
Department of Electrical Engineering
University of Queensland
St. Lucia, Australia

Stephen J. Dollinger, Ph.D.
Professor and Director of Clinical Training
Department of Psychology
Southern Illinois University at Carbondale
Carbondale, Illinois

Mervyn J. Eadie, M.D., Ph.D., F.R.C.P., F.R.A.C.P.
Roche-Utah Professor of Neurology and
  Neuropharmacology
Department of Medicine
University of Queensland
Royal Brisbane Hospital, Australia

Frederick T. Fraunfelder, M.D.
Chairman
Department of Ophthalmology
The Oregon Health Sciences Center
Portland, Oregon

Kelley B. Gelb
Krupnick, Campbell, Malone, and Roselli
  Law Offices
Fort Lauderdale, Florida

Bruce Hocking, D.P.H., D.I.H., F.A.C.O.M., F.R.A.C.G.P., M.F.O.M., M.A.R.P.S.
Director, Occupational Medicine
Corporate Human Resources
Telecom Australia
Melbourne, Victoria, Australia

Jon E. Krupnick
Krupnick, Campbell, Malone, and Roselli
  Law Offices
Fort Lauderdale, Florida

David Mackerras, Ph.D.
Honorary Research Consultant
Department of Electrical Engineering
University of Queensland
St. Lucia, Australia

Martha Meyer, B.S.
Senior Research Associate
Department of Ophthalmology
The Oregon Health Sciences Center
Portland, Oregon

R. P. F. Parkes, M.B., B.Med.Sc., F.R.A.C.P.
Director of Intensive Care
North West Regional Hospital
Burnie, Tasmania, Australia

Stuart P. Pegg, M.B.B.S., F.R.C.S.(Eng),
F.R.A.C.S., F.R.A.C.M.A.
Director of Surgery, and Director of the
  Burns Unit
Royal Brisbane Hospital
and Director of the Burns Unit
Royal Childrens Hospital
Brisbane, Australia

B. Raphael, Ph.D.
Head of Department
Department of Psychiatry
University of Queensland
and Director of Psychiatric Services
Royal Brisbane Hospital
Brisbane, Australia

H. J. ten Duis, M.D., Ph.D.
Associate Professor and Surgeon
Department of Traumatology
University Hospital
Groningen, The Netherlands

Jon D. Uman
Sellars, Supran, Cole, Marion, and Espy
  Law Offices
West Palm Beach, Florida

Martin A. Uman, M.A., Ph.D.
Professor and Chairman
Department of Electrical Engineering
University of Florida
Gainesville, Florida

Stuart P. Pegg, M.B.B.S., F.R.C.S.(Eng), F.R.A.C.S., F.R.A.C.M.A.
Director of Surgery, and Director of the
  Burns Unit
Royal Brisbane Hospital
and Director of the Burns Unit
Royal Childrens Hospital
Brisbane, Australia

B. Raphael, Ph.D.
Head of Department
Department of Psychiatry
University of Queensland
and Director of Psychiatric Services
Royal Brisbane Hospital
Brisbane, Australia

H. J. ten Duis, M.D., Ph.D.
Associate Professor and Surgeon
Department of Traumatology
University Hospital
Groningen, The Netherlands

Jon D. Uman
Sellars, Supran, Cole, Marion, and Espy
  Law Offices
West Palm Beach, Florida

Martin A. Uman, M.A., Ph.D.
Professor and Chairman
Department of Electrical Engineering
University of Florida
Gainesville, Florida

CONTRIBUTORS

**Christopher J. Andrews, B.E.(Hons),
M.Eng.Sc., Dip.Comp.Sc.,
M.B.B.S.(Hons), M.A.C.S., S.M.I.R.E.E.,
S.M.I.E.E.E.**
formerly Lecturer and Research Fellow
Department of Electrical Engineering
University of Queensland
St. Lucia, Australia
currently House Medical Officer
The Wesley Hospital
Brisbane, Australia
and medical practitioner in private practice

LaV. Bergstrom, M.D.
Professor of Surgery
Division of Head and Neck Surgery
Department of Surgery
University of California, Los Angeles

R. Cash, M.D.
Psychiatrist
Child and Family Therapy Unit
Royal Childrens Hospital
Brisbane, Australia

Mary Ann Cooper, M.D., F.A.C.E.P.
Associate Professor and Residency
  Research Director
Program in Emergency Medicine
University of Illinois Hospital
Chicago, Illinois

**Mat Darveniza, F.T.S., B.E., Ph.D.,
D.Eng., F.I.E.Aust., F.I.E.E.E.**
Professor in Electrical Engineering
  (Personal Chair)
Department of Electrical Engineering
University of Queensland
St. Lucia, Australia

Stephen J. Dollinger, Ph.D.
Professor and Director of Clinical Training
Department of Psychology
Southern Illinois University at Carbondale
Carbondale, Illinois

**Mervyn J. Eadie, M.D., Ph.D., F.R.C.P.,
F.R.A.C.P.**
Roche-Utah Professor of Neurology and
  Neuropharmacology
Department of Medicine
University of Queensland
Royal Brisbane Hospital, Australia

Frederick T. Fraunfelder, M.D.
Chairman
Department of Ophthalmology
The Oregon Health Sciences Center
Portland, Oregon

Kelley B. Gelb
Krupnick, Campbell, Malone, and Roselli
  Law Offices
Fort Lauderdale, Florida

**Bruce Hocking, D.P.H., D.I.H.,
F.A.C.O.M., F.R.A.C.G.P., M.F.O.M.,
M.A.R.P.S.**
Director, Occupational Medicine
Corporate Human Resources
Telecom Australia
Melbourne, Victoria, Australia

Jon E. Krupnick
Krupnick, Campbell, Malone, and Roselli
  Law Offices
Fort Lauderdale, Florida

David Mackerras, Ph.D.
Honorary Research Consultant
Department of Electrical Engineering
University of Queensland
St. Lucia, Australia

Martha Meyer, B.S.
Senior Research Associate
Department of Ophthalmology
The Oregon Health Sciences Center
Portland, Oregon

**R. P. F. Parkes, M.B., B.Med.Sc.,
F.R.A.C.P.**
Director of Intensive Care
North West Regional Hospital
Burnie, Tasmania, Australia

CONTENTS

Chapter 1

LIGHTNING — THE MYTHOLOGY PERSISTS

M. A. Cooper and C. J. Andrews

TABLE OF CONTENTS

Lightning has played a prominent part in almost all ancient religions and has a great deal of mystery and mythology surrounding it to this day, both because it is difficult to study and because it is so wondrous and awe inspiring when it occurs

I. RELIGION

Even the earliest peoples saw lightning as a powerful force. Lightning could not only destroy, but could also protect and warm a person by providing a source for fire before people learned to start and propagate fire at will.

Some primitive peoples characterized lightning as an animal or bird, including the American Indian, the Bantu of South Africa, and the Aborigine of western Australia. Witch doctors and magic men from various cultures were believed to have power to allay storms and to call on the gods to deliver water to their people or destruction to their enemies. They often used charms and potions made of wood, stones, or plants that were connected to lightning in their belief systems to cause harm, bring about favorable outcomes, or cure disease.

Lightning appears prominently in the Buddhist, Druidic, and ancient Egyptian religions. It was used by Jove, Jupiter, and Thor to express their power and often their anger in the ancient Greek, Roman, and Norse religions, respectively. Priests used storms and lightning as omens to interpret the wishes of the gods and control matters of state. Even in Judaic and Christian writings, it was seen as a sign of a superior being's presence, being noted several times in the Old Testament. In the middle ages, church bells were rung to break up thunderstorms and avert lightning. Churches were felt to be protected by God and were sometimes used for munitions storage, with spectacular explosions on more than one occasion. Uman[1] draws attention to the fact that the fifth day of the week must have been particularly important. The Anglo-Saxon Thursday is derived from the Norse Thor's day and has equivalence in the Danish Thorsday, the German Donnerstag (thunder day), and the Italian Giovedi (Jove's Day).

The Second International Conference on Lightning and Static Electricity (Oklahoma, 1988) chose the mystical thunderbird as its emblem. A modern automobile also uses the name of Thunderbird, so one can see that the feeling of power from lightning is still important to our culture.

Such is the penetration of these beliefs that the reports of the strike to York Minster, where the cathedral was struck the day before the enthronement of one of England's most controversial bishops, even today betray a superstitious belief in omens and warnings from the Deity.

II. SCIENCE

Aristotle, Socrates, and Pliny all made observations about lightning. Herodotus and, more recently, da Vinci also described lightning phenomena, but without defining it further. It remained for Benjamin Franklin, the "Father of Electricity", to determine that lightning was a form of electricity and to do many simple but elegant experiments that helped to define some of the basic properties of lightning and electricity. Franklin's "invention" of the lightning rod, which to this day remains almost unmodified, may have been the first practical application derived from the study of electricity.

More recently, it has been postulated that lightning may have had a part in the formation of life as we know it on earth. Urey and Miller suggest that lightning catalyzed the original linking of water, hydrogen, and nitrogen (in the form of ammonia and methane) into amino and nucleic acids, the building blocks of organic life, and carried out experiments that seem to support their hypothesis.

Medical knowledge regarding the pathophysiology of lightning injury was unformed until Critchley's pioneering work in 1932, although Jex-Blake began some early work in 1913. This theme is elaborated elsewhere in the volume.

Chapter 1

LIGHTNING — THE MYTHOLOGY PERSISTS

M. A. Cooper and C. J. Andrews

TABLE OF CONTENTS

III. MODERN MYTHOLOGY

Despite all that we know about lightning, there are still many myths that surround it. Probably the most common belief is that injuries from lightning are rare and, when they occur, are invariably fatal. While the incidence of lightning injuries varies by the part of the world and the topography of the land, they are quite common in many areas. Between 150 and 200 deaths from lightning are reported each year in the U.S., with a much larger number of nonfatal injuries occurring.

In their reviews of the medical literature, Cooper[2] and Andrews et al.[3] have shown that lightning injuries are fatal in only 20 to 30% of the cases, depending on how the data are analyzed. Given that usually only the most serious or "special-interest" cases are reported in the literature, extrapolation of these reports suggests that there are probably a minimum of 600 to 1200 injuries per year in the U.S. that often are of only minor degree. In a 2-week period in the summer of 1989, 21 persons in the Chicago area were involved in four different incidents, with only one death occurring. Lightning injuries are much more common in areas where there are large bodies of water (such as the Great Lakes, the Ohio, Mississippi, and Hudson river valleys, along the Atlantic coast, and in the Florida swamplands) than in desert areas or along the Pacific coast, although the western plains of the U.S. can provide wonderful lightning displays as well. Mountainous areas tend to have a greater number of lightning strikes and injured persons than flatlands.

Another myth could be called the "crispy critter" myth: the idea that when lightning strikes a victim they are burned to a crisp, vaporized, or reduced to a tiny pile of dust. Whenever one lectures on lightning, as the audience warms to the question-and-answer period, someone will invariably ask with a slightly embarrassed expression whether lightning is responsible for the stories told about persons walking down the street who burst into flames without apparent cause. Fortunately, the idea of vaporization and spontaneous combustion is the figment of several science fiction writers' and sensationalists' imaginations and has no basis in fact.

However, many quite reasonable and intelligent people believe that anyone hit by lightning will be severely burned, perhaps beyond recognition and repair, because of lightning's tremendous energy and violence. Fortunately, lightning seldom causes deep burns, but usually results in very superficial damage to the skin and soft tissues, although it may play havoc with the cardiac and neurological systems as it interferes severely with the body's natural electrical circuits. While burns from lightning can occasionally mimic the burns seen with high-voltage electrical injuries, this is quite rare, probably because of the brief time course involved in a strike.

Mystery and fantasy still surround lightning. One of the sensationalist rumor sheets sold at the checkout line in many grocery and drug stores in the U.S. recently reported the story "Lightning Turns Man into Woman". One might understand how lightning could result in emasculation and a necessary switch to the female sex if a part of the "crispy critter" myth were operational, but it is difficult to understand how lightning could turn a woman anatomically, physiologically, or genetically into a man.

Many persons who might otherwise have survived their lightning injuries have died because bystanders believed that the victim was "electrified" by the strike and could electrocute the rescuers if they attempted to aid the victim. While lightning energy can spread through the surface of the ground and backflash through pipes, wires, and other metal objects, this happens in a few hundredths of a second and the lightning energy does quickly dissipate and will not harm anyone who would touch the victim.

However, a victim who has been hit by lightning may be in an area that continues to be dangerous during a thunderstorm, since lightning can and often does strike the same place twice (despite the popular belief to the contrary). It is only logical that if conditions favor a lightning strike occurring once, lightning may strike again under the same conditions. For instance, tall buildings are struck many times each year, and sometimes in a single thunderstorm, which is one reason that properly designed lightning protection systems are so important. Thus, it is prudent not to subject a rescuer to excess risk in this manner, and removal of a victim from a risk area in accord with the usual practice of first aid is wise, but not for the reason of residual electrification!

A notion that continues to occur in the medical literature is that lightning causes a state of "suspended animation", so that a lightning victim can recover from a prolonged cardiac or respiratory arrest without any brain damage. The initial report on which this belief is based cited a pediatric case that did not have a documented prolonged arrest. In addition, the original report claimed that the child recovered from the arrest (the management of which included open chest cardiac massage) with an IQ higher than that tested prior to the injury, which is difficult to accept. There have been other anecdotal reports similar to this, but there exists no experimental evidence for believing that a lightning victim who receives prolonged cardiopulmonary resuscitation will be protected from hypoxic brain damage or will have their mental abilities improved by the lightning stroke. The preponderance of evidence is quite contrary to this and in agreement with the current literature on cardiac arrest.

Some people believe that the victim will be spared cardiac damage if the lightning travels over the right side of the body (thus "avoiding" the heart, which is thought to be on the "left" side of the body). Lightning energy may "flash over" the exterior of the victim's body, markedly decreasing the cardiac insult. Alternatively, lightning energy may penetrate the body. Electrical energy treats the soft tissues of the body like a continuous medium, although it does have a tendency to travel through the areas of the body that offer the least resistance, especially the blood vessels. These pathways lead readily to the heart. Even if the energy did flow over only one side of the body, a cursory study of human anatomy shows the heart to be situated in the center of the chest, extending into both sides with only a slight preponderance into the left chest, so that it would be affected regardless of the "side" struck.

Other myths concern the degree of protection a person has if they are inside a building. Unfortunately, there are multiple reports of persons being injured by flow of current through plumbing, telephones, electrical appliances, or other conduits, although they are within a building. Small open-sided sheds, tents, and soft-top automobiles all offer substantial risk to the person caught in a violent thunderstorm.

Many people believe that rubber, in the form of tires or shoe soles, is a good insulator against lightning. Since lightning can traverse a mile or more of air, which is a much better insulator than rubber, an inch or less of rubber (or more likely a petroleum by-product) cannot be counted on to protect a person. The recommendation that persons take off the raincoat they are wearing and place it on the ground to insulate themselves in a storm is even more ludicrous.

Lightning, as a spectacular natural phenomenon, has had a large mythology generated about it. Many "modern myths" have hampered not only effective resuscitation of lightning victims, but also research in this area.

REFERENCES

1. **Uman, M. A.,** *The Lightning Discharge,* Academic Press, Orlando, FL, 1987.
2. **Cooper, M. A.,** Lightning injuries, in *Management of Wilderness and Environmental Emergencies,* Auerbach, P. et al., Eds., Macmillan, New York, 1983.
3. **Andrews, C. J., Darveniza, M., and Mackerras, D.,** Lightning injury — a review of clinical aspects, pathophysiology, and treatment, *Adv. Trauma,* 4, 241, 1989.

Chapter 2

PHYSICS OF LIGHTNING

Martin A. Uman

TABLE OF CONTENTS

I. INTRODUCTION

In this chapter, we examine those aspects of lightning important to an understanding of lightning injury and death. We first discuss the characteristics of lightning and then consider briefly the mechanisms by which that lightning causes damage, injury, and death. A more detailed discussion of the electrical aspects of lightning events is found in Chapter 3.

II. HOW MUCH LIGHTNING IS THERE?

Brooks,[1] in 1925, on the basis of worldwide weather station data on the occurrence of thunder, estimated that the global lightning flash rate, both cloud and ground discharges, was about 100/s. Modern measurements made with satellites[2-4] are in reasonably good agreement with this early estimate. A global flash rate of 100/s represents a global flash density, the number of lightning flashes per unit area per unit time, of about 6 per square kilometer per year (km^{-2} yr^{-1}), which would appear reasonable considering the data on flash density over land to be presented next and the fact that there is less lightning over the oceans than over the land.

Prentice[5] has summarized much of the published and unpublished data on average lightning flash density. For example, southeast Queensland, Australia has a total (cloud and ground discharges) flash density of 5 km^{-2} yr^{-1}, of which 1.2 km^{-2} yr^{-1} are ground flashes; Norway, Sweden, and Finland have measured ground flash densities between 0.2 and 3 km^{-2} yr^{-1}, depending on location; and South Africa has ground flash densities from below 0.1 to about 12 km^{-2} yr^{-1}, depending on location. Flash density maps and the statistics noted above are given by Prentice and Mackerras[6] and Mackerras[7] for Australia, by Muller-Hillebrand[8] for Scandinavia, and by Anderson[9] and Anderson and Eriksson[10] for South Africa.

Piepgrass et al.[11] measured the total (cloud and ground discharges) flash density at the Kennedy Space Center in Florida during the months of June and July, 1974 through 1980. Total flash densities ranged from 3.7 km^{-2} mo^{-1} in 1977 to 21.9 km^{-2} mo^{-1} in 1975. The mean of 6 years was 12 km^{-2} mo^{-1}, with a standard deviation of 8 km^{-2} mo^{-1}. From the ratio of cloud flashes to ground flashes reported by Livingston and Krider,[12] Piepgrass et al.[11] estimate a mean ground flash density of 4.6 km^{-2} mo^{-1}, with a standard deviation of 3.1 km^{-2} mo^{-1}.

Maier et al.[13] mapped geographic variations of flash density in south Florida. Their results show that, due to local meteorological effects that occur along the Florida coastline, flash density may vary by an order of magnitude over distances from the coastline inland 20 to 30 km. Most of the lightning occurs inland due to the effect of the sea breeze in producing storms there, and relatively little occurs along the coastline. Darveniza and Uman,[14] in the Tampa Bay area of Florida, found that the ground flash density, averaged over 2 years, determined from seven CIGRE 10-kHz flash counters was between 7 and 17 flashes km^{-2} yr^{-1}, depending on the assumptions made about the effective range and counter response to cloud flashes. A CIGRE 500-Hz counter, based on the extrapolation of 4 months of summer measurement and with an effective range and cloud flash response determined in Australia, gave a yearly ground flash density of 9.5. A two-station magnetic direction finding system operated only during the summer months gave an extrapolated yearly ground flash density of 12.9 ± 5.2 km^{-2} yr^{-1}.

Ground flash density has, until the recent development of sophisticated lightning location systems such as the magnetic direction finding networks used by Maier et al.[13] and by Darveniza and Uman,[14] not been considered a simple parameter to measure. The thunderday level, the number of days per month or year on which thunder is heard, is more easily measurable and hence has been recorded at most weather stations worldwide for many years. A world thunderday map is found in Figure 1, and a thunderday map of the U.S. is given in Figure 2. A considerable effort has been made to relate the thunderday level, for which there are considerable statistics, to the flash density, for which there is relatively little, since it is a knowledge of the

Chapter 2

PHYSICS OF LIGHTNING

Martin A. Uman

TABLE OF CONTENTS

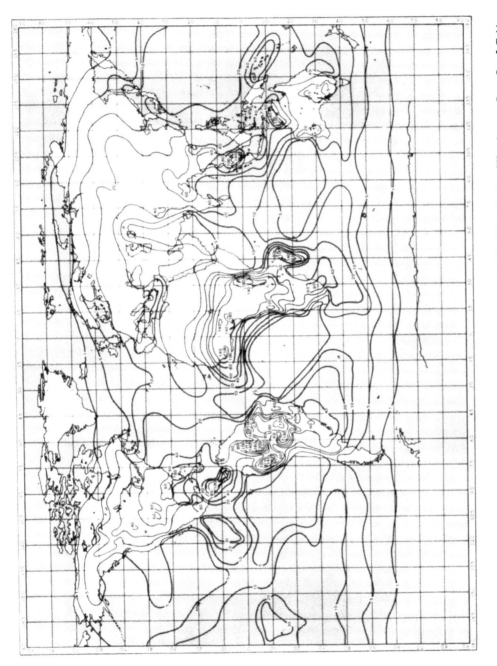

FIGURE 1. World Thunderday Map. Mean annual days with thunderstorms. (Adapted from *World Distribution of Thunderstorm Days, Part 2. Tables of Marine Data and World Maps*, World Meteorological Organization Publ. 21, Geneva, Switzerland, 1956.)

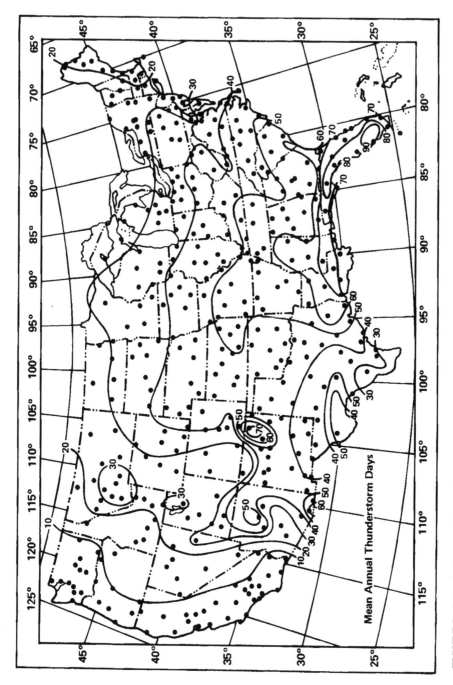

FIGURE 2. A thunderday map of the U.S. compiled from data from 450 air weather stations shown as dots. Most stations had 30-year records and all had at least 10-year records. (Adapted from MacGorman, D. R., Maier, M. W., and Rust, W. D., Lightning Strike Density for the Contiguous United States from Thunderstorm Duration Records, NUREG/CR-3759, Office of Nuclear Regulatory Research, U.S. Nuclear Regulatory Commission, Washington, D.C., May 1984.)

flash density that is important in the assessment of the lightning hazard. Prentice[5] has reviewed 17 proposed relations between these two parameters. Most are of the form

$$N_g = aT_D^b \text{ km}^{-2} \text{ yr}^{-1} \tag{1}$$

where N_g is the ground flash density, T_D the annual thunderdays, and a and b are empirical constants. Typically, a = 0.1 to 0.2 and b = 1. The only measurements of statistical significance are from South Africa and Australia. Anderson[9] and Anderson and Eriksson[10] review measurements made with 120 flash counters located throughout South Africa, where the annual thunderday level varied from about 3 to about 100 and where the ground flash density ranged from below 0.1 to about 12 km^{-2} yr^{-1}. The relation that best fits the South African data is

$$N_g = 0.023 \; T_D^{1.3} \text{ km}^{-2} \text{ yr}^{-1} \tag{2}$$

although for a given T_D, N_g can vary by a factor up to about 5 from the value of N_g in Equation 2. Mackerras,[7] in Australia, made measurements with 26 counters in a region where the flash density varied from about 0.2 to 3.0 km^{-2} yr^{-1} and the annual thunderday level from about 10 to about 100. His data are best fit by the expression

$$N_g = 0.01 \; T_D^{1.4} \text{ km}^{-2} \text{ yr}^{-1} \tag{3}$$

where for a given T_D, N_g varies by a factor of about 2 from the value of N_g found in Equation 3.

It might be expected that the exponent b in Equation 1 would exceed unity since the higher number of thunderdays, the longer one might expect the storms to last on each day. If this be true, the flash density should correlate more linearly with the number of thunderhours than with the number of thunderdays and, indeed, there is some evidence that this is the case.[5,15] MacGorman et al.[15] have determined the following relation between ground flash density and thunderhours T_H,

$$N_g = 0.054 \; T_H^{1.1} \text{ km}^{-2} \text{ yr}^{-1} \tag{4}$$

Since both the number of thunderhours or thunderdays per year and the flash density vary from year to year, both parameters must be measured over many years for the relationship of average flash density to average thunderhours or thunderdays to be statistically meaningful. Anderson et al.[16] recommend taking data for at least 11 years, one solar cycle, although Freier[17] finds little evidence for coupling between solar activity and thunderstorms.

As an illustration of potential problems in relating ground flash density to thunderstorm days, Ishii et al.[18] point out that near Sakata, Japan, where there are about the same number of thunderstorm days (13) in winter as in summer, the ground flash density varies an order of magnitude between the two seasons, being about 0.4 km^{-2} for the 4 summer months and 0.05 km^{-2} for the 4 winter months.

III. THE SOURCES OF LIGHTNING

Most studies of cloud electric fields and charges have been concerned with the cloud type called cumulonimbus, also referred to as the thundercloud or thunderstorm, the primary producer of lightning. There have, however, been some measurements of the electrical properties of stratus, stratocumulus, cumulus, nimbostratus, altocumulus, and altostratus clouds,[19] and of the electric fields and the charge on precipitation at ground level from nonthunderstorm rain, sleet, and snow.[20] Any of the cloud types listed above can potentially produce lightning or some related form of electrical discharge, as can snowstorms (which are apparently similar to cumulonimbus in charge structure) and the clouds above volcanoes and due to other turbulent environments such as dust storms.

A model for the charge structure of a typical thundercloud was developed by the early 1930s. The model was derived from ground-based measurements of both the electric fields associated with the static cloud charges and the electric field changes associated with the effective neutralization of a portion of those cloud charges by lightning.[14-21] In the model, the primary thundercloud charges form a positive electric dipole, i.e., a positive charge region P containing charge Q_P located above a negative charge region N containing charge Q_N, as shown in Figure 3. By the end of the 1930s, Simpson and Scrase[25] had verified the existence of this fundamental dipole structure from in-cloud measurements made with instrumented balloons, and, additionally, had identified a localized region of positive charge Q_P at the base of the cloud, as is also illustrated in Figure 3.

Subsequent measurements of cloud electric fields made both inside and outside the cloud have confirmed the general validity of the double-dipole charge structure.[26-32] A fundamental problem, however, in developing an essentially static cloud charge model is that neither the fields nor the charges that produce them are really steady in time. Among other effects, there are substantial rapid field changes due to lightning and subsequent slower field recoveries. Illustrating these effects are the records of the electric field vs. time at ground near thunderstorms found, for example, in Jacobson and Krider.[36]

The overall charge associated with the negative charge region is thought not to be uniformly distributed, but, rather, localized in pockets of relatively high space-charge concentration. Evidence for this localized charge concentration is found in the fact that individual return strokes in a multiple-stroke ground flash tap different negative charge regions. Krehbiel et al.[37] found that the negative charge regions discharged by individual strokes to ground were displaced primarily horizontally from one other. The charge locations found in New Mexico, Florida, and Japan by the same research group are illustrated in Figure 4. Apparently, the negative charge region contributing to ground discharges is located in the same relatively narrow temperature range, roughly -10 to -25°C, for storms in these very different environments.

Recent reviews of the charge generation and separation processes postulated to occur in cumulonimbus clouds have been given by Magono,[38] Latham,[39] Lhermitte and Williams,[40] Illingworth,[41] and Williams.[42] According to Mason,[43] an adequate theory of thunderstorm electrification must account for the fact that the mature stage of a thunderstorm of moderate intensity is characterized by lightning, strong vertical air motion, and the presence of precipitation; that it lasts for about 30 min, during which time the average current (negative charge downward) is about 1 A; that the first lightning usually occurs within 20 min of the formation of precipitation; that the basic electrical structure is a positive dipole; that the location of negative charge is near -5°C; and that there is an association of field growth with the development of soft hail. Latham[39] finds this list still "largely acceptable" in light of recent research, which he reviews, and adds the condition that electric fields of magnitude near 4×10^5 V/m be generated within the central regions of the thunderstorm within about 20 min of the formation of precipitation. The presence of soft hail, as specified by Mason,[43] plays a prominent role in the electrification processes favored by Latham,[39] but is not necessary to some of the other theories.

Basically, there are two types of theories for the generation of the main cloud charge dipole: (1) precipitation theories and (2) convection theories. The former are viewed in the literature as the more significant, but both types could well play some part in cloud electrification. We now consider each of these types of theories.

In the precipitation theories, heavy, falling precipitation particles interact with lighter particles carried in updrafts. The interaction process serves to charge the heavy particles negatively and the light particles positively, after which gravity and updrafts separate the

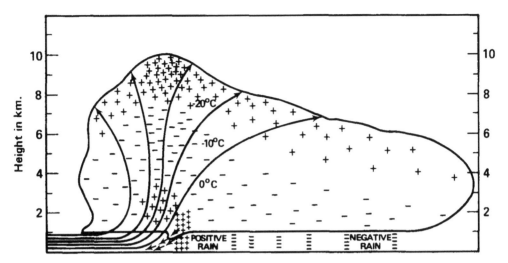

FIGURE 3. A diagram showing the distribution of air currents and electrical charge in a typical convective thunderstorm in England inferred by Simpson and Scrase[25] from instrumented balloon flights. A summary of the charge locations found in this study and in a later study reported by Simpson and Robinson[26] is given in Simpson and Robinson's Table 3. (From Simpson, G. and Scrase, F. J., *Proc. R. Soc. London Ser. A*, 161, 309, 1937. With permission.)

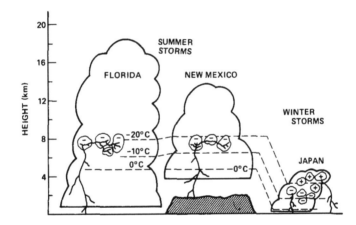

FIGURE 4. Drawing illustrating the altitude and distribution of ground-flash charge sources observed in summer thunderstorms in Florida and New Mexico and winter thunderstorms in Japan as determined from simultaneous measurement of the electric field at a number of ground stations by Krehbiel et al.[73] Note the positive lightning shown in the winter thunderstorm, a common feature of that type of storm. (From Krehbiel, P. R. et al., in *Proceedings in Atmospheric Electricity*, Ruhnke, R. H. and Latham, J., Eds., Deepak, Hampton, Virginia, 1983, 408. With permission.)

opposite charges to form a positive cloud dipole. Charge transfer can be by collision in which two initially uncharged precipitation particles become, after collision, oppositely charged, as, e.g., in collisions between hail and ice crystals, the presently preferred mechanism for thunderstorm electrification;[44-46] or by induction in which two uncharged but electrically polarized (one sign of charge on the top, the other sign on the bottom due to the ambient field) precipitation particles collide in such a way that the small light hydrometeor absorbs charge from the bottom of the larger heavy precipitation particle, as the lighter particle moves upward.[47] The induction process serves to enhance the initial field in which it operates. Kuettner et al.[48] discuss the relative importance of inductive and noninductive interaction mechanisms in thunderstorm electrification. Individual hydrometeors may also acquire charges in the process of melting or freezing, or by the capture or release of free ions or charged aerosol particles.[46]

In the convective electrification theories, charge which has been accumulated near the earth's surface or across regions of varying air and cloud conductivity, including the so-called screening layer at the cloud boundary, is moved in bulk to the observed locations by the air flow associated with the thunderstorm.[49-53] Magono[38] provides an interesting discussion of the arguments for and against convective theories. Perhaps related to the argument for the existence of convective electrification is Magono's review of the observations of lightning in clouds whose tops do not reach the freezing level, so-called warm-cloud lightning. If such observations are accepted as true, precipitation-charging mechanisms involving collisions between different forms of ice or between ice and supercooled water are not necessary for electrification, although this certainly does not rule out the possibility that they occur and even that they are the dominant charging mechanism in the usual thunderstorm. Williams[42] reviews a variety of reasons why a precipitation mechanism alone is insufficient to account for the available observations of thunderstorm electrification and hence why a convective mechanism could play an important role in charge separation.

The small positive charge region at the base of the cloud may not be present in all thunderstorms, or it may simply be well localized and hence relatively difficult to detect.[26] The positive charge could be produced by one or more of the following proposed mechanisms: (1) a mechanism similar to those postulated for producing the primary dipole charges, e.g., by hailstones falling through a cloud of supercooled droplets and ice crystals at temperatures between 0 and -20°C, as suggested by Jayaratne and Saunders[54] on the basis of laboratory experiments (see also References 55 and 56); (2) the release of positive corona at the ground and its subsequent upward motion to the cloud base, as suggested by Malan and Schonland[57] and Malan;[28] or (3) the deposition by lightning, as suggested by Marshall and Winn.[31]

IV. TYPES OF LIGHTNING

Lightning is a transient, high-current electric discharge whose path length is measured in kilometers and whose most common source, as we have discussed, is the electric charge separated in ordinary thunderstorm clouds (cumulonimbus). Well over half of all lightning discharges occur within the thunderstorm cloud and are called intracloud discharges. The usual cloud-to-ground lightning (sometimes called streaked or forked lightning) has been studied more extensively than other lightning forms because of its practical interest (e.g., as the cause of injuries and death, disturbances in power and communication systems, and the ignition of forest fires) and because lightning channels below cloud level are more easily photographed and studied with optical instruments. Cloud-to-cloud and cloud-to-air discharges are less common than intracloud or cloud-to-ground lightning. All discharges other than cloud-to-ground are often lumped together and called cloud discharges.

Berger[58] has categorized lightning between the cloud and earth in terms of the direction of motion, upward or downward, and the sign of charge, positive or negative, of the leader which initiates the discharge. That categorization is illustrated in Figure 5. Category 1 lightning is the most common cloud-to-ground lightning. It accounts for over 90% of the worldwide cloud-to-ground flashes, perhaps over 99%, accurate worldwide statistics being unavailable. It is initiated by a downward-moving negatively charged leader, as shown, and hence lowers negative charge to earth. Category 3 lightning is also initiated by a downward-moving leader, but the leader is positively charged, and hence the discharge lowers positive charge. Less than 10% of the worldwide cloud-to-ground lightning is of this type. Category 2 and 4 lightning is initiated by leaders which move upward from the earth and are sometimes called ground-to-cloud discharges. These upward-initiated discharges are relatively rare and generally occur from mountain tops and tall, man-made structures. Category 2 lightning has a positively charged leader and may lead to the lowering of negative cloud charge; Category 4 has a negatively charged leader and may lead to the lowering of positive cloud charge. In the next section, we discuss Category 1 lightning in some detail, since it is the type of lightning about which most is known, and then briefly consider Category 3 lightning.

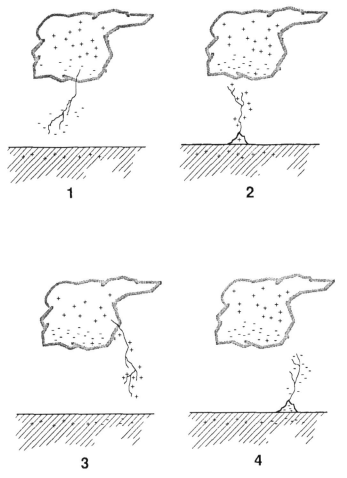

FIGURE 5. Types of lightning according to Berger. (From Berger, K., *Bull. Schweiz. Elektrotech. Ver.*, 69, 353, 1978. With permission.)

V. CLOUD-TO-GROUND LIGHTNING

A still photograph of a negative cloud-to-ground discharge is shown in Figure 6. This Category 1 discharge starts in the cloud and eventually brings to earth tens of coulombs of negative cloud charge. The total discharge is termed a *flash* and has a time duration of about half a second. A flash is made up of various discharge components, among which are typically three or four high-current pulses called *strokes*. Each stroke lasts about a millisecond, the separation time between strokes being typically several tens of milliseconds. Lightning often appears to "flicker" because the human eye can just resolve the individual light pulse associated with each stroke.

In the idealized model of the cloud charges shown in Figures 3, 4, and 5, the main positive and negative charge regions, called P and N, respectively, are of the order of many tens of coulombs of positive and negative charge, respectively, and the lower *p* region contains a smaller positive charge. The following discussion of negative cloud-to-ground lightning is illustrated in Figure 7. The *stepped leader* initiates the first *return stroke* in a flash by propagating from cloud to ground in a series of discrete steps. The stepped leader is itself initiated by a *preliminary breakdown* within the cloud, although there is disagreement about the exact form and location of this process. In Figure 7, the preliminary breakdown is shown in the lower part of the cloud between the N and P regions. The preliminary breakdown sets the stage for negative charge to

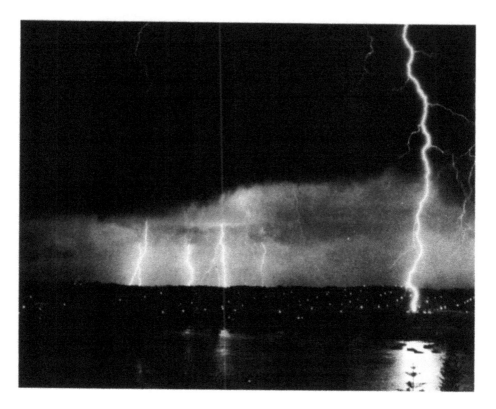

FIGURE 6. Photograph of negative cloud-to-ground lightning.

be lowered toward ground by the stepped leader. Photographically observed leader steps are typically 1 μs in duration and tens of meters in length, with a pause time between steps of about 50 μs. A fully developed stepped leader lowers up to 10 or more C of negative cloud charge toward ground in tens of milliseconds with an average downward speed of about 2×10^5 m/s. The average leader current is in the 100 to 1000-A range. The steps have pulse currents of at least 1 kA. Associated with these currents are electric- and magnetic-field pulses with widths of about 1 μs or less and risetimes of about 0.1 μs or less. The stepped leader, during its trip toward ground, branches in a downward direction, producing the downward-branched geometrical structure seen in Figures 6 and 7.

The electric potential of the bottom of the negatively charged leader channel with respect to ground has a magnitude in excess of 10^7 V. As the leader tip nears ground, the electric field at sharp objects on the ground or at irregularities of the ground itself exceeds the breakdown value of air, and one or more upward-moving discharges are initiated from those points, thus beginning the *attachment process*. An understanding of the physics of the attachment process is central to an understanding of the operation of ground-based lightning protection and the effects of lightning on humans and animals, since it is the attachment process that determines where the lightning attaches to objects on the ground and the value of the early currents which flow. When one of the upward-moving discharges from the ground (or from a lightning rod or an individual) contacts the downward-moving stepped leader, some tens of meters above the ground, the leader tip is connected to ground potential, the voltage level of the upward-moving leader since it is attached to ground. The leader channel is then discharged when a ground potential wave, the first *return stroke,* propagates continuously up the previously ionized and charged leader path. The upward speed of a return stroke near the ground is typically one third to one half the speed of light, and the speed decreases with height. The total transit time from ground to the top of the channel is of the order of 100 μs. The first return stroke produces a peak current near ground of typically 35 kA, with a time from zero to peak of a few microseconds. Currents measured at the

15

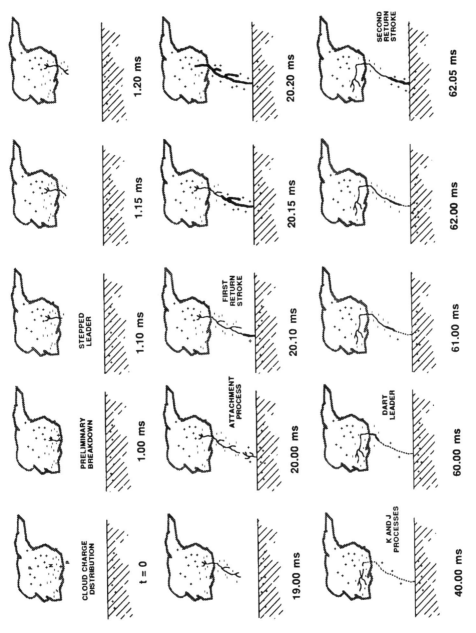

FIGURE 7. A drawing illustrating some of the processes involved in negative cloud-to-ground lightning, Category 1. (From Uman, M. A., *The Lightning Discharge*, Academic Press, London, 1987. With permission.)

ground fall to half of the peak value in about 50 μs, and currents of the order of hundreds of amperes may flow for times of a few milliseconds up to several hundred milliseconds. The larger-lasting currents are known as *continuing current*. The rapid release of return stroke energy heats the leader channel to a temperature near 30,000K and generates a high-pressure channel which expands and creates the shock waves which eventually become thunder. Additional discussion on thunder is found in the next section. The return stroke effectively lowers to ground the charge originally deposited on the stepped leader channel and initiates the lowering of other charge which may be available to the top of its channel.

After the return stroke current has ceased to flow, the flash, including charge motion in the cloud, may end. The lightning is then called a single-stroke flash. On the other hand, if additional charge is made available to the top of the channel, a continuous *dart leader* may propagate down the residual first-stroke channel at a speed of about 3×10^6 m/s. During the time between the end of the first return stroke and the initiation of a dart leader, *J*- and *K-processes* occur in the cloud. There is controversy as to whether these processes are necessarily related to the initiation of the dart leader. The dart leader lowers a charge of the order of 1 C by virtue of a current of about 1 kA. The dart leader then initiates the second (or any subsequent) return stroke. Some leaders begin as dart leaders, but toward the end of their trip toward ground become stepped leaders. These leaders are known as dart-stepped leaders and have different ground termination points (and upward leaders) from the first stroke. Dart leaders and return strokes subsequent to the first are usually not branched. Dart-leader electric-field changes typically have a duration of about 1 ms. Subsequent return-stroke overall field changes are similar to, but usually a factor of two or so smaller than, first return-stroke field changes. Subsequent return-stroke currents have faster zero-to-peak rise times than do first-stroke currents, but similar maximum rates of change.

The time between successive return strokes in a flash is usually several tens of milliseconds, as we have noted in the first paragraph of this section, but can be tenths of a second if a continuing current flows in the channel after a return stroke. Continuing current magnitudes are of the order of 100 A and represent a direct transfer of charge from cloud to ground. The typical electric-field change produced by a continuing current is linear for roughly 0.1 s and is consistent with the lowering of about 10 C of cloud charge to ground. Between one fourth and one half of all cloud-to-ground flashes contain a continuing current component. Continuing current is not illustrated in Figure 7.

Positive cloud-to-ground flashes, those lowering positive charge, though relatively rare, are of considerable practical interest because their peak current and total charge transfer can be much larger than the more common negative ground flash. The largest recorded peak currents, those in the 200 to 300-kA range, are due to the return strokes of positive lightning. Positive flashes to ground are initiated by leaders which do not exhibit the distinct steps of their negative counterparts. Rather, they show a luminosity which is more or less continuous but modulated in intensity. Positive flashes are generally composed of a single stroke followed by a period of continuing current. Positive flashes are probably initiated from the upper positive charge in the thundercloud when that cloud charge is horizontally separated from the negative charge beneath it. Positive flashes are relatively common in winter thunderstorms (snow storms), which produce few flashes overall, and are relatively uncommon in summer thunderstorms. The fraction of positive lightning in summer thunderstorms apparently increases with increasing latitude and with increasing height of the ground above sea level.

The material on cloud-to-ground discharges found in this section was abstracted primarily from Uman.[59]

VI. THUNDER

Thunder, the acoustic radiation associated with lightning, is sometimes divided into the categories "audible", sounds that one can hear, and "infrasonic", below a few tens of hertz, a frequency range that is inaudible. This division is made because it is thought that the mechanisms that produce audible and infrasonic thunder are different. Audible thunder is thought to be due to the expansion of a rapidly heated return stroke channel,[60-62] as noted in the previous section, whereas infrasonic thunder is thought to be associated with the conversion to sound of the energy stored in the electrostatic field of the thundercloud when lightning rapidly reduces that cloud field.[63-65]

The best available measurements of thunder overpressure, energy, and frequency spectra are due to Holmes et al.[66] They observed ground flash thunder spectra to exhibit a mean peak value of acoustic power at 50 Hz with a mean total acoustic energy of 6.3×10^6 J. About 0.2% of the estimated input energy to ground flashes was converted to distant thunder. The thunder measured by Holmes et al.[66] far from the lightning represents the superposition of the sound from many sources, each source being a short section of the return stroke channel. The details of the energy input to short channel sections and resultant formation of an outward-moving shock wave have been modeled by Hill,[62] Plooster,[67] Jones et al.[68] Troutman,[69] and Colgate and McKee.[63] Overpressures of the order of 4 or 5 atmospheres are predicted at about 5 cm from the channel and about 1 or 2 atmospheres at 10 cm. Clearly, these overpressures are sufficient to cause damage to the human eardrum and perhaps other human functions in the event of a direct or very close strike to that human.

VII. MECHANISMS FOR LIGHTNING DAMAGE

A. GENERAL EFFECTS

The amount and type of lightning damage an object suffers is due to both the characteristics of the lightning discharge and the properties of the object. The physical characteristics of lightning of most interest are the currents, the electromagnetic fields including the optical and ultraviolet portion of the spectrum, and the acoustic wave.

Four properties of the lightning current can be considered important in producing damage: (1) the peak current, (2) the maximum rate of change of current, (3) the integral of the current over time (i.e., the charge transferred), and (4) the integral of the current squared over time, the so-called action integral. Let us examine each of these properties and the type of damage that it can produce.

For objects that present a resistive impedance, such as a ground rod driven into the earth, a human or an animal, a long power line, or a tree, the peak voltage on the object relative to ground will be proportional to the peak current, i.e., $V = IR$, where V is the voltage in volts, I the current in amperes, and R the object's resistance in ohms (see also Appendix to Chapter 3). For example, a 50,000-A current injected into a 400-Ω power line produces a line voltage of 20 million V. Such large voltages lead to electric discharges from the struck object to the ground through the air, or through or across insulating materials. These flashovers can, for example, short circuit a power system or kill people who are standing close to an object, such as a tree, that is struck. Discharges which occur from a struck object are referred to as *side flashes*. In the next section, we will examine the details of a lightning strike to a human or an animal, including the effects of side flashes. The magnetic forces produced by the peak lightning currents are large and can crush metal tubes and pull wires from walls.

For objects that have an inductive impedance, such as wires between electronic systems or in an electronic system, the peak voltage will be proportional to the maximum rate of change of the lightning or lightning-induced current ($V = L \, di/dt$, where L is the object's inductance in henries). For example, if 1 m of wire has an inductance L of 10^{-6} H and carries a typical rate-of-rise of lightning current of $di/dt = 10^{11}$ A/s, 100,000 V is generated across the wire. Thus, a small fraction of the peak lightning current can easily cause damage to solid-state electronic devices via the generation of inductive voltage differences.

The heating or burn through of metal sheets such as airplane wings, space vehicle surfaces, or metal roofs is, to first approximation, proportional to the lightning charge transferred (average current times time). Generally, large charge transfers are due to long-duration (tenths of a second to seconds) lightning currents in the 100 to 1000-A range, i.e., continuing current, rather than to larger currents that have a relatively short duration.

The heating of many solid objects and the explosion of insulators is, to first approximation, due to the value of the action integral. In the case of wires, the action integral represents the heat that is generated by the resistive impedance of the wire. About 1% of negative strokes to ground have action integrals exceeding 10^6 A²-s. About 5% of positive strokes have action integrals exceeding 10^7 A²-s. In the case of most insulators, this heat vaporizes the internal material and the resultant gas pressure causes an explosive fracture.

Two properties of the radio frequency (rf) electromagnetic fields are sufficient to describe most of the important damage effects: (1) the peak value of the field and (2) the maximum rate of rise to this peak. For certain types of antennas or metal exposed to the lightning rf field, the peak voltage on the metal is proportional to the peak field. These antennas are commonly referred to as capacitively coupled. For other antennas, such as a loop of wire in an electronic circuit or an underground communication cable, the peak voltage is proportional to the maximum rate of change of the field. The degree of coupling of fields through holes or apertures in metal skins of, e.g., aircraft and spacecraft is generally proportional to the rate of change of the electromagnetic fields.

The optical and ultraviolet portion of the lightning electromagnetic output can cause temporary blindness in humans and animals as well as permanently affect vision and cause cataracts.[70] The shock wave produced by a flash can, at close range, break windows and eardrums.[71]

B. APPLICATION TO HUMANS AND ANIMALS, OUTDOORS AND INDOORS

In addition to the hazards from close lightning noted above — blindness, acoustic shock, and side flash — an additional hazard from nearby lightning is due to so-called *step voltage*. Step voltage is due to a voltage difference between two places on the earth's surface as the result of the injection of current in the earth from the nearby lightning stroke. Step voltages appear between the legs of a human or animal, driving potentially harmful current into the body. The magnitude of the step voltage V can be determined from the expression

$$V = \frac{I}{2\pi\sigma}\left(\frac{1}{d} - \frac{1}{d+s}\right) = \frac{I}{2\pi\sigma}\left(\frac{s}{d(d+s)}\right)$$

where I is the lightning current in amperes, σ the earth conductivity in mhos/m, s the distance between the legs in meters in the direction of the lightning strike, and d the distance between the point of lightning strike and the near leg in meters.

Assuming a lightning current of 20 kA, a soil conductivity of 10^{-2} mhos/m, a step length of 0.5 m, and a distance to the strike point of 10 m, the step voltage becomes 1.5 kV. The internal resistance of a current path through both legs is probably of the order of 100 Ω, which means that the current through the legs will reach near or over 10 A. For humans, this current does not generally reach the heart or respiratory center and hence probably will not result in permanent injury or death, but for four-legged animals such as horses and cows it can reach the heart, and such events lead to a significant number of animal deaths each year. From the equation given above, the peak step voltage is directly proportional to the peak current and, when d is greater than s, roughly inversely proportional to the square of the distance from the lightning to the person.

Berger[72] has discussed the details of a lightning strike to a person. When a person is directly struck by lightning or encounters the lightning current via a side flash, the resulting potential difference across the body is so high that generally the skin is punctured at the points of current entry and exit. Let us assume the lightning strike is to the head of a person. Then the top and bottom of the body are punctured and an increasing current flows through the body. At this point, either internal breakdown can occur through the body in the form of a high current arc or the major lightning current may discharge via surface flashover. A large gap in air between metal electrodes suffers electrical breakdown at an average electric field intensity near 500 kV/m. Through the human body or across a wet surface, the value may be as low as 200 kV/m (see Chapter 3). If the person is about 2 m tall, an external flashover can therefore be expected to occur when the potential is between 400 and 1000 kV. In the absence of an internal discharge, when the head-to-foot body resistance is taken as about 1000 Ω, the current in the person can, at the instant of external flashover, reach as much as 1000 A (1000 kV/1000 Ω), a value still far below the typical first-stroke peak current of 35 kA. If external flashover takes place, as is apparently most often the case, an electric arc is established in the air across the body. Such an arc has an axial electric field of about 2 kV/m. Thus, the potential difference across the body collapses to 4.0 kV (2 kV/m × 2 m), and the current through the person becomes about 4 A (4.0 kV/1000 Ω), a value which will be maintained until the current in the lightning discharge ceases. The interior of the human body will therefore be subjected to a short-duration current peak reaching just over 1000 A within some 10 µs, followed by a constant current of the order of 5 A maintained for several milliseconds. Much larger currents flow across the skin and can burn the skin, melt metal jewelry, and literally blow off clothes and shoes by virtue of the steam generated from rain and perspiration on the skin. If instead of external flashover, an internal discharge occurs, considerably more life-threatening damage will occur. The circumstances of internal flashover are discussed in detail in Chapter 3. If the unfortunate person is struck by several lightning strokes in one flash, the process just described can be repeated several times. The tens-of-microsecond period before the first-stroke current peak will be preceded by the 100 A-level current due to the upward connecting leader which serves to determine the strike point. An individual can be involved in an upward leader which does *not* connect with the downward leader. Such an event is certainly less hazardous, due to its short duration and relatively low current, than a direct strike and is a likely cause, along with step voltage, for the simultaneous electrical shocking of large groups of people.

Finally, it should be noted that lightning injury and death, while most common outdoors, can certainly occur indoors. The mechanism is side flash. The usual source is the telephone, although any systems such as electrical appliances or water pipes which connect to substantial metal outside the structure can be a source of side flash. In the case of the telephone, a voltage difference is generated between the person and the telephone, either because the telephone wires outside are directly struck or have relatively large voltages induced by close strikes, or because the potential of earth, power ground, or other grounds attached to the person are raised due to lightning current injection into them, and the resulting voltage difference between the headset and the body causes a spark between the headset and the ear, often burning the ear canal and breaking the eardrum, sometimes causing death, as discussed in Appendix 1 and elsewhere in this book. Such a spark can occur in typical telephones when the potential of the telephone relative to that of the ear exceeds about 10 kV. These effects are discussed in more detail in Chapter 3.

REFERENCES

1. **Brooks, C. E. P.,** The distribution of thunderstorms over the globe, *Geophys. Mem.,* 13, 147, 1925.
2. **Orville, R. E.,** Global distribution of midnight lightning — September to November 1977, *Mon. Weather Rev.,* 109, 391, 1981.
3. **Kotaki, M., Kuriki, I., Kotoh, C., and Sugiuchi, H.,** Global distribution of thunderstorm activity observed with ISS-B, *J. Radio Res. Lab.,* 28, 49, 1981.
4. **Turman, B. N. and Edgar, B. C.,** Global lightning distributions at dawn and dusk, *Geophys. Res.,* 87, 1191, 1982.

5. **Prentice, S. A.,** Frequency of lightning discharges, in *Lightning,* Vol. 1, Golde, R. H., Ed., Academic Press, New York, 1977, 465.

6. **Prentice, S. A. and Mackerras, D.,** Recording range of a lightning-flash counter, *Proc. Inst. Electr. Eng.,* 116, 1969.

7. **Mackerras, D.,** Prediction of lightning incidence and effects in electrical systems, *Electr. Eng. Trans.,* 14, 73, 1978.

8. **Muller-Hillebrand, D.,** Lightning-counter measurements in Scandinavia, *Proc. Inst. Electr. Eng.,* 112, 203, 1965.

9. **Anderson, R. B.,** Lightning research in southern Africa, *Trans. S. Afr. Inst.,* 71, 3, 1980.

10. **Anderson, R. B. and Eriksson, A. J.,** Lightning parameters for engineering application, *Electra,* 69, 65, 1980.

11. **Piepgrass, M. V., Krider, E. P., and Moore, C. B.,** Lightning and surface rainfall during Florida thunderstorms, *J. Geophys. Res.,* 87, 11,193, 1982.

12. **Livingston, J. M. and Krider, E. P.,** Electric fields produced by Florida thunderstorms, *J. Geophys. Res.,* 83, 385, 1978.

13. **Maier, M. W., Boulanger, A. G., and Sax, R. I.,** An Initial Assessment of Flash Density and Peak Current Characteristics of Lightning Flashes to Ground in South Florida, NUREG/CR-1024, U.S. Nuclear Regulatory Commission, Office of Standards Development, Washington, D.C., September 1979.

14. **Darveniza, M. and Uman, M. A.,** Research into lightning protection of distribution systems II — results from Florida field work 1978 and 1979, *IEEE Trans. PAS,* 103, 673, 1984.

15. **MacGorman, D. R., Maier, M. W., and Rust, W. D.,** Lightning Strike Density for the Contiguous United States from Thunderstorm Duration Records, NUREG/CR-3759, U.S. Nuclear Regulatory Commission, Office of Nuclear Regulatory Research, Washington, D.C., May 1984.

16. **Anderson, R. B., Van Niekerk, H. R., Prentice, S. A., and Mackerras, D.,** Improved lightning flash counters, *Electra,* 66, 85, 1979.

17. **Freier, G. D.,** A 10-year study of thunderstorm electric fields, *J. Geophys. Res.,* 83, 1373, 1978.

18. **Ishii, M., Kawamura, T., Hojyo, J., and Iwaizumi, T.,** Ground flash density in winter thunderstorm, *Res. Lett. Atmos. Electr.,* 1, 105, 1981.

19. **Imyanitov, I. M., Chubarina, Ye V., and Shvarts, Ya M.,** Electricity in clouds: technical translation from Russia, NASA TT F-718, 1972.

20. **Simpson, G. C.,** Atmospheric electricity during disturbed weather, *Geophys. Mem.,* 84, 1, 1949.

21. **Wilson, C. T. R.,** On some determinations of the sign and magnitude of electric discharges in lightning flashes, *Proc. R. Soc. London Ser. A,* 92, 555, 1916.

22. **Wilson, C. T. R.,** Investigations on lightning discharges on the electric field of thunderstorms, *Philos. Trans. R. Soc. London Ser. A,* 221, 73, 1920.

23. **Appleton, E. V., Watson-Watt, R. A., and Herd, J. F.,** Investigations on lightning discharges and on the electric fields of thunderstorms, *Proc. R. Soc. London Ser. A,* 221, 73, 1920.

24. **Schonland, B. F. J. and Craib, J.,** The electric fields of South African thunderstorms, *Proc. R. Soc. London Ser. A,* 114, 229, 1927.

25. **Simpson, G. and Scrase, F. J.,** The distribution of electricity in thunderclouds, *Proc. R. Soc. London Ser. A,* 161 309, 1937.

26. **Simpson, G. C. and Robinson, G. D.,** The distribution of electricity in the thunderclouds, XI, *Proc. R. Soc. London Ser. A,* 177, 281, 1941.

27. **Kuettner, J.,** The electrical and meteorological conditions inside thunderclouds, *J. Meteorol.,* 7, 322, 1950.

28. **Malan, D. J.,** Les descharges dans l'air et la charge inferieure positive d'un nuage orageux, *Ann. Geophys.,* 8, 385, 1952.

29. **Huzita, A. and Ogawa, T.,** Charge distribution in the average thunderstorm cloud, *J. Meteorol. Soc. Jpn.,* 54, 285, 1976.

30. **Winn, W. P., Moore, C. B., and Holmes, C. R.,** Electric field structure in an active part of a small, isolated thundercloud, *J. Geophys. Res.,* 86, 1187, 1981.

31. **Marshall, T. C. and Winn, W. P.,** Measurements of charged precipitation in a New Mexico thunderstorm: lower positive charge centers, *J. Geophys. Res.,* 87, 7141, 1982.

32. **Taniguchi, T., Magono, C., and Endoh, T.,** Charge distribution in active winter clouds, *Res. Lett. Atmos. Electr.,* 2, 35, 1982.

33. **Weber, M. E., Christian, H. J., Few, A. A., and Stewart, M. F.,** A thundercloud electric field sounding: charge distribution and lightning, *J. Geophys. Res.,* 87, 7158, 1982.

34. **Weber, M. E., Stewart, M. F., and Few, A. A.,** Corona point measurements in a thundercloud at Langmuir Laboratory, *J. Geophys. Res.,* 88, 3907, 1983.

35. **Byrne, G. J., Few, A. A., and Weber, M. E.,** Altitude, thickness and charge concentration of charged regions of four thunderstorms during TRIP 1981, based upon *in situ* balloon electric field measurements, *Geophys. Res. Lett.,* 10, 39, 1983.

36. **Jacobson, E. A. and Krider, E. P.**, Electrostatic field changes produced by Florida lightning, *J. Atmos. Sci.*, 33, 113, 1976.
37. **Krehbiel, P. R., Brook, M., and McCrory, R.**, An analysis of the charge structure of lightning discharges to the ground, *Geophys. Res.*, 84, 2432, 1979.
38. **Magono, C.**, *Thunderstorms*, Elsevier, Amsterdam, 1980.
39. **Latham, J.**, The electrification of thunderstorms, *Q. J. R. Meteorol. Soc.*, 107, 277, 1981.
40. **Lhermitte, R. and Williams, E.**, Cloud electrification, *Rev. Geophys. Space Sci.*, 21, 984, 1983.
41. **Illingworth, A. J.**, Charge separation in thunderstorm: small scale processes, *J. Geophys. Res.*, 90, 6026, 1985.
42. **Williams, E. R.**, Large-scale charge separation in thunderclouds, *J. Geophys. Res.*, 90, 6013, 1985.
43. **Mason, B. J.**, A critical examination of theories of charge generation in thunderstorms, *Tellus*, 5, 446, 1953.
44. **Reynolds, S. E., Brook, M., and Gourley, M. F.**, Thunderstorm charge separation, *J. Meteorol.*, 14, 426, 1957.
45. **Caranti, J. M. and Illingworth, A. J.**, Surface potentials of ice and thunderstorm charge separation, *Nature*, 284, 44, 1980.
46. **Illingworth, A. J.**, Charge separation in thunderstorm: small scale processes, *J. Geophys. Res.*, 90, 6026, 1985.
47. **Sartor, J. D.**, The role of particle interactions in the distribution of electricity in thunderstorms, *J. Atmos. Sci.*, 224, 601, 1967.
48. **Kuettner, J. P., Leven, Z., and Sartor, J. D.**, Thunderstorm electrification-inductive or non-inductive?, *J. Atmos. Sci.*, 38, 2470, 1981.
49. **Grenet, G.**, Essai d'expication de la charge electrique des nuages d'orages, *Ann. Geophys.*, 3, 306, 1947.
50. **Grenet, G.**, Le nuage d'orage: machine electrostatique, *Meteorologie*, I-53, 45, 1959.
51. **Vonnegut, B.**, Possible mechanism for the formation of thunderstorm electricity, *Bull. Am. Meteorol. Soc.*, 34, 378, 1953.
52. **Vonnegut, B.**, Possible mechanism for the formation of thunderstorm electricity, *Geophys. Res.*, 42, 169, 1955.
53. **Wagner, P. B. and Telford, J. W.**, Charge dynamics and electric charge separation mechanism in convective clouds, *J. Rech. Atmos.*, 15, 97, 1981.
54. **Jayaratne, E. R. and Saunders, C. P. R.**, The rain gush, lightning and the lower positive charge center in thunderstorms, *J. Geophys. Res.*, 89, 11,816, 1984.
55. **Marshall, T. C. and Winn, W. P.**, Comments on "the rain gush", lightning, and the lower positive center in thunderstorms, by E. R. Jayaratne and C. P. R. Saunders, *J. Geophys. Res.*, 90, 10,753, 1985.
56. **Jayaratne, E. R. and Saunders, C. P. R.**, Thunderstorm electrification: the effect of cloud droplets, *J. Geophys. Res.*, 90, 13,063, 1985; reply, *J. Geophys. Res.*, 90, 10,753, 1985.
57. **Malan, D. J. and Schonland, B. F. J.**, The distribution of electricity in thunderclouds, *Proc. R. Soc. London Ser. A*, 209, 158, 1951b.
58. **Berger, K.**, Blitzstrom-parameter von Aufwartsblitzen, *Bull. Schweiz. Elektrotech. Ver.*, 69, 353, 1978.
59. **Uman, M. A.**, *The Lightning Discharge*, Academic Press, London, 1987.
60. **Few, A. A.**, Power spectrum of thunder, *J. Geophys. Res.*, 74, 6926, 1969.
61. **Few, A. A.**, Acoustic radiations from lightning, in *Handbook of Atmospherics*, Vol. 2, Volland, H., Ed., CRC Press, Boca Raton, FL, 1981.
62. **Hill, R. D.**, Channels heating in return stroke lightning, *J. Geophys. Res.*, 76, 637, 1971.
63. **Colgate, S. A. and McKee, C.**, Electrostatic sound in clouds and lightning, *J. Geophys. Res.*, 74, 5379, 1969.
64. **Dessler, J.**, Infrasonic thunder, *J. Geophys. Res.*, 78, 1889, 1973.
65. **Few, A. A.**, The production of lightning-associated infrasonic acoustic sources in thunderclouds, *J. Geophys. Res.*, 90, 6175, 1985.
66. **Holmes, C. R., Brook, M., Krehbiel, P., and McCrory, R.**, On the power spectrum and mechanism of thunder, *J. Geophys. Res.*, 76, 2106, 1971.
67. **Plooster, M. N.**, Numerical model of the return stroke of the lightning discharge, *Phys. Fluids*, 14, 2124, 1971.
68. **Jones, D. L., Goyer, G. G., and Plooster, M. N.**, Shock wave from a lightning discharge, *J. Geophys. Res.*, 73, 3121, 1968.
69. **Troutman, W. S.**, Numerical calculation of the pressure pulse from a lightning stroke, *J. Geophys. Res.*, 74, 4595, 1969.
70. **Fraunfelder, F. and Meyer, M.**, Ocular system, in *Lightning Injuries: Electrical, Medical, and Legal Aspects*, Andrews, C. J., Cooper, M. A., Darveniza, M., and Mackerras, D., Eds., CRC Press, Boca Raton, FL, 1992, chap. 6, sect. VI.
71. **Kristensen, S. and Tveteras, K.**, Lightning induced acoustic rupture of the tympanic membrane, *J. Laryingol. Otol.*, 99, 711, 1985.
72. **Berger, K.**, Blitzforschung and personen-blitzschutz, *Elektrotech. Z.*, ETZ-A, 92, 1971.
73. **Krehbiel, P. R., Brook, M., Lhermitte, R. L., and Lennon, C. L.**, Lightning charge structure in thunderstorms, in *Proceedings in Atmospheric Electricity*, Ruhnke, R. H. and Latham, J., Eds., Deepak, Hampton, VA, 1983, 408.

Chapter 3

ELECTRICAL ASPECTS OF LIGHTNING INJURY AND DAMAGE

Mat Darveniza

TABLE OF CONTENTS

I. INTRODUCTION

The effects of lightning currents can only be understood by considering the electrical aspects of their flow through an object. This requires the development of electrical circuit models of the stricken object and an analysis of the distribution of current, voltage, and energy absorption throughout the object. Further, the magnitude of the lightning current through a stricken object depends on the interaction between it and the physical system which delivers the current to it. Therefore, an electrical circuit model of the lightning stroke is also required. If there is a direct strike to the object, the lightning stroke can be described as a simple current source. If the lightning strikes some distance away, then electrical circuit models of the intervening physical system are required to determine the indirect effects of the lightning on the object of concern. These matters are considered in this chapter, and enable the various effects of lightning currents to be examined in a realistic and systematic manner.

II. ELECTRICAL CIRCUIT MODELS

Electrical circuits[1] can be developed to model the flow of electrical current through an object. The conducting and insulating components are modeled by resistors of appropriate values. In circumstances where currents and voltages vary with time, it is also often necessary to include inductors and capacitors in the circuit models. These components constitute impedances to current flow, and determine the distributions of voltage, current, and energy absorption throughout the object.

The simplest circuit models are those which only consider resistors. Good conductors are modelled by low-valued resistors ($<1\ \Omega$), poor conductors by medium-valued resistors (1 to about $100,000\ \Omega$) and insulators by high-valued resistors. The resistors may be arranged in series circuits, in parallel circuits, or in series-parallel combinations. Analyses of series and parallel circuits are given in an appendix to this chapter, and these enable the determination of voltages, currents, and energy absorption using the appropriate equations in the appendix.

The simplest resistors are those which conform to Ohm's law,

$$v(t) = Ri(t) \tag{1}$$

The resistance R is determined by the component's physical characteristics of resistivity, cross-sectional area, and length. The resistance is often thought of as a constant, and indeed it is for ohmic resistors at constant temperature. But all resistors exhibit temperature dependence. For some, the metallic conductors and resistors, the resistance increases with temperature. For others, such as ionic conductors, semiconductors, and insulators, the resistance decreases with temperature. This negative temperature dependence of resistance is of crucial importance when considering the flow of current in parallel pathways. As described in the appendix, it can lead to a concentration of most of the current in one pathway, and can give rise to what is called runaway thermal breakdown of the resistive path.

Other resistors exhibit nonlinear characteristics and do not conform to Ohm's law. Typically, an increase of voltage causes a greater than proportional increase of current. These are the nonlinear resistors. An extreme form of nonlinearity occurs when the voltage developed across a resistor becomes large enough to cause electrical breakdown. This takes the form of an electrical discharge either through or over the surface of the (previously sound) resistor, and the resultant arc is usually characterized by a large current, a low arc voltage, and a high arc current temperature. Nonlinear resistors are also considered in the appendix, including their tendency to promote thermal runaway when connected in parallel.

Lightning currents and voltages are, of course, time varying, and so it is often necessary to include inductive and capacitive effects in the electric circuit models. It is shown (in the appendix) that inductive effects can cause high voltages for circuits subjected to currents with high rates of rise, and that capacitive currents can be significant with high rates of rise of voltage.

While homogeneous objects can be modeled by simple electrical circuits, quite complex circuits are often required to model nonhomogeneous objects. The complexity of the circuit model necessarily increases when a number of objects has to be considered as part of a system of objects subjected to a lightning strike. The analysis of the strike incident often focuses on a specific component, e.g., determination of the amount of current and therefore the energy absorbed. There is a particularly powerful technique in electrical circuit theory for such a specific analysis. This is Thévenin's theorem. It is described in the appendix, and in later sections in this chapter. Thévenin equivalent circuits are used to determine the expected magnitudes of lightning currents that flow through a body.

III. THE LIGHTNING STROKE AS A CURRENT SOURCE

It is generally accepted that the return strokes of a lightning flash can be modeled as an "ideal" current source.[2] This means that the magnitude of the current delivered to a stricken object can be considered independent of its resistance; referring to the equivalent circuit given as Figure 3b (in the appendix), $I \approx I_s$ when $R_{th} >> R_b$. From an electrical viewpoint, R_{th} is the surge impedance of the stroke channel, and it is generally considered to be greater than $1000 \, \Omega$. Most stricken objects have a resistance of much less than $1000 \, \Omega$; if the resistance is not initially small, electrical breakdown will soon make it so (remember Uman's example in Chapter 2 — a 50,000-A current through a 400-Ω resistance produces a voltage of 20 million V, which would certainly cause breakdown).

This raises the question of "how much voltage is associated with a lightning stroke?". The theoretical answer is found in the voltage equivalent circuit of Figure 2a. Consider an average stroke current (I_s) of 30,000 A and a surge impedance (R_{th}) of $2000 \, \Omega$. Then, a fair estimate of the "open-circuit" voltage (V_{th}) is 60 million V. From a practical point of view, the interest is only in the voltage developed after contact is made to a stricken object, and lightning current flows through it. This voltage is calculated using the appropriate one of Equations 1, 4, or 10.

A. THE DIRECT STRIKE

All the current in a lightning flash is delivered to the stricken object "in the field". The characteristics of lightning currents are detailed in Chapter 2. Of course, if the resistance of the stricken body is not small, external flashover may occur and much of the current will discharge over its external surface rather than pass through it internally. Fortunately, while lightning flashes to ground can be quite frequent, it is an uncommon event for a normal-sized object to be struck "in the field".

B. INDUCED SURGES

The voltages induced on a conductor by a nearby lightning strike to ground are small compared with those arising from a direct strike to it. The largest voltages are those induced on conductors above the ground. There is a considerable body of literature, theoretical and experimental,[4] which shows that the voltages induced by lightning on overhead lines very rarely exceed 200,000 V, and are mostly in the range of 10,000 to 50,000 V. As will be discussed below, the associated surge currents are also small compared with those in a direct strike.

C. PROPAGATION OF LIGHTNING ALONG ELECTRICAL LINES

Electrical power and telephone lines are connected to nearly all buildings. These lines can act both as "collectors" of lightning and as "conductors" of the resulting surges to the buildings. Because such lines are well distributed spatially, the frequency of lightning surges reaching buildings is very much greater than the frequency of direct strikes. Fortunately, their severity is very much less (but can still be hazardous).

Consider, first of all, electrical lines which are above ground — the so-called overhead lines. Lightning can impose surges on them either by direct strike or by induction from lightning strikes to nearby ground. Whatever the mechanism, the maximum voltage which can propagate along the line is limited by the capacity of its electrical insulation to carry the voltage without electrical flashover to ground. The insulation level depends on the type of line — it can be as high as 1 million V for a high-voltage power line and as low as 10,000 V for low-voltage and telephone lines. This limits the magnitude of the current which such a surge can deliver to an object connected to the line (i.e., an object subjected to a lightning surge after propagation along a line). The appropriate Thévenin equivalent is Figure 3a, in which R_{th} is now the surge impedance of the line; typically, R_{th} is 250 to 500 Ω. It follows, therefore, that the maximum current which can be delivered by a line-connected lightning surge is 8000 A ($2 \times 1,000,000/250$ — the factor of 2 is a multiplier due to a transients phenomenon). Much smaller surge currents are more likely, typically 400 to 800 A (associated with surge voltages of 50,000 and 100,000 V). Clearly, and most importantly from damage and injury viewpoints, these surges are far less severe than those associated with a direct strike.

The severity becomes even less if the electrical lines are buried in the ground, so-called underground power and telephone cable.[4] There are several reasons for this: the ground shields the cable (at least in part) from the full lightning current, and the surge "leaks" into the earth as it propagates along the cable.

There are, however, two situations which can cause severe surges to reach an object after propagation along a line. The first arises if the lightning strike is close by, e.g., if an overhead line is struck just one or two spans away (say 25 to 100 m), most of the current in the lightning flash might flow into the building if it has a good earth (resistance less than 10 Ω). The second can occur if the lightning flash is nearby and if the electrical resistivity of the surrounding earth is high (say, greater than 500 Ω-m). In this circumstance, even underground cables can deliver large surge currents into a building.

D.   EARTH POTENTIAL RISE (EPR)

When lightning strikes the ground or an object on the ground, the current flows away from the stricken point to the surrounding earth. Because the earth has a finite electrical resistivity and because of the resistance of the connection to ground, significant voltage is developed at the strike point with respect to remote earth potential.

The resistance (R_e) of the connection to earth, usually called the "earth" resistance, depends on the resistivity of the surrounding earth and on the type, number and dimensions of the earthing electrodes. Usually, Equation 1 is used to calculate the EPR, but even a simple calculation soon shows the need for a more complex model. Consider an average lightning current of 30,000 A passing through an earth resistance of 20 Ω. The EPR is 600,000 V, and such a voltage will surely cause ionization and sparking in the surrounding soil. The resulting nonlinearity makes Equation 4 applicable, and the net effect is to lower the effective resistance of the connection to earth. This so-called lightning surge reduction of the earth resistance has been studied extensively (see, for example, Reference 2), and it is quite common to find the effective resistance to be as low as one fifth of that which would be measured at low currents with conventional instruments.

Notwithstanding the ameliorating influence of nonlinearity, EPR can still be dangerously large (e.g., 100 kA and 5 Ω gives 500,000 V). Inductive effects should also be accounted for using Equation 10, making EPR even larger. Further, all objects close to the stricken object will be raised in voltage with respect to remote earth. If there is present a conductive connection to a remote earth, a large voltage difference can appear between the stricken object and this connection. Two likely situations of potential hazard come readily to mind. Consider a person in a building, which is either struck directly by lightning, or which discharges through its earth a substantial portion of the current in a nearby lightning strike. If the person is using electrical equipment (such as a telephone) connected via an electrical line to a remote earth (such as at a transformer or telephone exchange earth), that person may be exposed to a hazardous surge voltage. Of necessity, and referring to Figure 2a, the Thévenin resistance of the source will be small (being that of the earth resistance), and so the resulting current is only limited by the resistance of the body R_b. A similar situation occurs if a person external to the stricken building touches it. That person is also exposed to much of the EPR of the stricken building.

Both of the above situations can be described as "touch"-voltage hazards. But there is also a "step"-voltage hazard to people or animals near an object struck by lightning. The lightning current flows into the earth away from the stricken point and establishes concentric lines of equipotentials around it. For a simple connection to earth, the difference in potential between two adjacent points separated by a distance s and at a radius d from the stricken point, i.e., the step voltage (V_{st}), is dependent on the current magnitude (I), and the soil resistivity (ρ), as well as on d and s (see Chapter 2). Again, the Thévenin equivalent circuit of Figure 3a is used to calculate the current through a body of resistance R_b caused by V_{st} (as before, R_b dominates). For any given incident (a particular I and ρ), the potential hazard (V_{st} and I_b) depends both on the radial distance d and on the length of the step s. A person standing on one leg (or with both legs together) is safer than one in the act of a two thirds-m stride; obviously, it will be more hazardous for a large four-legged animal such as a horse or cow, particularly if it is facing the point of strike. This circumstance is the not uncommon event of injury to a person or animal standing near a tree struck by lightning.

E. THE SIDE FLASH

As already discussed, the flow of lightning currents through an object gives rise to voltages which can be calculated using Equation 10. If a body is close to the stricken object, as depicted in Figure 1, the developed voltage (V) may cause an electrical discharge between them. The magnitude of V and its dependence on I, di/dt, R, and L have already been considered, and of course may be large. For the circumstance shown in Figure 1, it is not dependent on the earth resistance (R_e); in other circumstances, it may be. The likelihood of a side flash is obviously also dependent on the air gap distance (d). A side flash may occur if the electrical stress on the air gap (V/d) exceeds about 500 kV/m. Again, the ensuing body current is determined using the Thévenin equivalent of Figure 3a, and as before, R_b usually dominates.

IV. THE EFFECTS OF LIGHTNING CURRENT FLOW ON STRICKEN OBJECTS

It is evident from the preceding section that the magnitude of the lightning current is very different for the direct strike event and for the other situations considered. These last can be called indirect events, and include induced surges, surges after propagation along electrical lines, touch and step surges and side flashes. For direct strikes, the currents can have magnitudes between 3 and 200 kA, whereas the currents caused by indirect surges will never exceed 8 kA, and will mostly be less, typically 400 to 800 A.

Clearly, the consequences of the two will be quite different. Both, however, depend on the manner by which the current enters and exits the stricken object, and on the magnitude and the distribution of the energy absorbed by the object as a result of the passage of current.

A. DIRECT STRIKES

There are many descriptions in the literature of the effects of lightning currents on trees, on wood and masonry, and soil. A very readable reference is Uman's book.[5] Most of the literature relates to effects on wood, in both living trees and the wood used in buildings and power line poles and crossarms.[6] The literature includes field observations of lightning strikes and laboratory studies with artificial lightning currents.

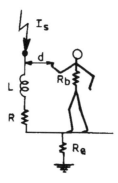

FIGURE 1. The circumstances for a side flash.

Trees and unseasoned wood poles contain a large amount of water. Typically, the moisture content is about 100% (expressed as the percentage of the oven-dry mass). Water is present in green wood in three forms — partly as free extracellular water in cell cavities and in pores and fibers; partly as intercellular water absorbed by the porous cellulose substance of the cell walls, and by chemical combination with the cellulose molecules. The dividing line is the fiber saturation moisture content of about 32%; all water above this moisture content is free.

There are many current pathways from the top of a tree or pole to ground. The internal pathways are the moisture-laden fibers and pores, and there are paths on or near the surface of the wood. The surface wood may be relatively dry (about 14% moisture content when in equilibrium with the surrounding air), or it may be wet by rain.

The electrical behavior of wood is dominated by this moisture — its overall content and its distribution throughout the wood. The resistance between the top of a living tree or a green pole and ground is at least 1000 Ω.[6,8] So a direct lightning strike, even with a small current, will cause sufficient voltage to cause breakdown and hence current discharge in a discrete arc column, either internally through the wood or externally over or near its surface. The reason for the discrete arc column is that the breakdown mechanism is the runaway thermal process or decaying resistor process described in the appendix for parallel resistors with negative temperature dependence. The blast effect of this discharge current concentrated in a discrete arc column is spectacular if confined inside the wood. Severe mechanical damage results because the wood is split violently. If the arc is on the surface, little or no damage occurs; if it is just below the surface, slivers of sapwood are gouged out.

Laboratory studies[6] have elucidated the mechanism of the blast damage. When an impulse current arc is confined in wood, the high temperature arc column is cooled by its exposure to the water in its vicinity (indeed, the arc will have been formed in one of the water-laden pores or fibers). Conduction is maintained by a high arc voltage, typically 40 kV for each meter length of wood (which is nearly two orders of magnitude larger than for an arc burning freely in air). The instantaneous power of the arc is enormous, e.g., 30,000 A for an average lightning stroke current flowing through a 10-m length of wood generates a power of 12,000 MW for the short time the current flows (tens of microseconds) — this is the output power of several large power stations. The energy is absorbed by the water in the wood; it is converted to high pressure steam, which first crushes the fiber walls surrounding the arc column and then splits the wood mechanically (a steam blast process). Usually, the shattered wood displays a clear "furrow", which indicates the location of the discharge current arc column. These "furrows" are often obvious in photographs;[5,6] the furrow diameter increases with increasing current magnitude.

It is evident, therefore, that the fate of a stricken tree or pole is determined by the location of the arc discharge path. If it is internal, severe damage results; if it is just below the surface, wood near the surface is gouged out; if it is on or just above the surface, little or no mechanical damage results.

Extensive laboratory studies[6] (with artificial lightning impulses) have been made of the factors which influence the location of the discharge arc path for wood poles and crossarms subjected to direct strikes with artificial lightning. The dominating influence is the moisture, its content, and its location. If the wood is green (i.e., has a high internal moisture content) and if an electrical connection is made to the moist internal wood, the arc path is internal whether the surface wood is dry or wet by rain. But if the moisture content is not high, the arc path is on the surface, particularly if the surface is rain wet. This tendency for a surface arc path is enhanced if the electrical connection to the pole is at the surface only, i.e., the discharge is required to find its own connection to the moist interior, and this is often prevented by the dry layers of wood just below its surface — a kind of insulating "skin".

Some numerical values of the electrical breakdown voltages for wood[6] will prove useful in later consideration of lightning strikes to people. Typically, dry and rain-wet seasoned poles and crossarms break down at stresses of 500 and 350 kV/m, respectively. Because the internal wood is dry, the breakdown path is either on or just under the surface, i.e., an external flashover path. If the wood is green, i.e., still retains most of the water in the previously living tree, the breakdown stresses can be as low as 150 to 250 kV/m. The breakdown path is always internal if the voltage is applied using a metal bolt or coachscrew which contacts the moist internal wood. The breakdown mechanism is the decaying resistor process. With such low internal breakdown stresses, external flashovers do not occur even if the external surface is wet by water. However, if the initially green wood is allowed to become partially seasoned (i.e., to dry out a little), external flashovers can occur at stresses of 200 to 300 kV/m if the electrical connection is at the surface only (e.g., a wire-wrap electrode). Even in this condition of surface flashover paths, the presence of an easy connection to the moist internal wood can cause a transition to an internal breakdown, e.g., a metal bolt or even a hole in the wood along the path of the flashover.

This fairly extensive account of direct lightning strikes to trees and green poles has been included because there are some intriguing parallels with the effects of direct strikes to people.

First, there is the matter of moisture content. About 60% of the mass of a human body is water, and about one third of this is extracellular.[9] Second, there are many parallel pathways for current flow inside the body and, of course, there are the surface pathways which may be significant if the body's surface or clothes are wet by perspiration or rain. It is generally accepted that the electrical resistance of the body is between 300 and 1000 Ω when the surface contact resistance is low. Therefore, a direct lightning strike, even with a small current, will produce enough voltage to cause electrical breakdown and hence current discharge internally through the body or over its surface. If internal, it is reasonable to expect that the thermal runaway (or decaying resistor) process will cause a discrete discharge with a high arc voltage, as for an arc confined inside wood. The high arc energy would be absorbed by converting the surrounding water to high-pressure steam, which would cause severe local damage to the surrounding tissue. The resulting blast effect can be expected to cause a "furrow" indicating where the discharge current flowed through the tissue. However, if the arc is on the skin surface, either because of surface wetness or because of metallic objects on the surface (such as a necklace, hand-held umbrella or golf club), little internal tissue damage will occur, although the surface arc may produce some superficial damage to skin tissue, and any arc-generated steam may "blow" off the person's clothes.

The parallels between lightning strikes to people and to green poles and trees are sufficiently intriguing to venture some further postulations. We have seen that the electrical stress required for discharge over a wet wood surface can be as low as 200 to 300 kV/m. It seems entirely reasonable to suppose the same is true for the moist surface of a human body. We have seen that the likelihood of an internal discharge path increases for a pole if there is a good electrical connection (such as a bolt) to the moist internal wood. Is it likely that there is a parallel in the case of the human body? Do such orifices as the mouth, eyes, or ears offer an easy portal for the entry of discharge currents into the body, particularly if the strike point is to the head and near one of these orifices?

The final matter to consider is the damage or burn injury that occurs at the entry and exit points of direct-strike lightning currents. There are two substantial reasons why the effects at these points can be expected to be exacerbated. The first is the direct exposure of tissue to current arcing through the air. Such an arc is at a high temperature (well over 2000°C), and it contains energetic ions which bombard and erode the surface with which it makes electrical contact. The second reason is the relatively high electrical resistance of the contact zone, comprising both contact resistance and constriction resistance. The total electrical circuit then comprises three resistors in series — two relatively high-valued resistances at the entry and exit points and the body resistance. As discussed in the appendix for series-connected resistors (see the numerical example), most of the voltage drops and most of the energy absorption are expected in the contact zones at the entry and exit points. Thus, these local areas would be subject to arcing and to high temperature rise, and these must cause localized damage and burns to tissue.

A related matter is the effect of metal jewelry on lightning current injuries. A conducting object of some length, such as a metal necklace, must influence the path of the discharge by intercepting and diverting the current. If the metal object has sufficient mass so that its electrical resistance is low, current flow through the object will not raise its temperature to a high level, but there will be entry and exit points for the current, with localized damage and burns as just described. If the object has little mass, and particularly if it has multiple links as in a chain necklace, the resulting high electrical resistance may cause multiple arcs or even complete fusion; then, burns and damage to the tissue would be expected at multiple points along the object.

B. INDIRECT SURGES

It has already been shown that the maximum prospective current due to an indirect lightning surge is 8000 A, and that more likely prospective currents are 400 to 800 A. The Thévenin equivalent circuit of Figure 3a provides the model for analyzing the expected currents.

In the section on direct strikes, it was seen that the human body can be considered to have two states with respect to the flow of lightning currents. First, there is the resistive state in which the conduction of current is mostly limited by the body resistance (R_b). Then there is the arc discharge state which occurs when the voltage (developed during the first resistive state) exceeds the electrical breakdown voltage, and therefore the discharge current flows in an arc column of very low resistance.

The extent of the damage to tissue and injury to the person must be totally dependent on whether or not the discharge arc state occurs. The electrical conditions which determine the state have already been identified, and it is now possible to consider the current flow effects.

1. Discharge Arc State

If the indirect surge applies a voltage in excess of about 200 kV to the body, electrical breakdown will occur, and the surge current will be discharged through an arc. The magnitude of the arc current is determined by the incident surge voltage and by the Thévenin impedance of the source (see Figure 3a). Whether the arc path is through the body or over its surface, the likely discharge currents are in the range of 400 to 8000 A. So significant damage and injury are likely if the arc is internal, as occurs with a direct lightning strike. If the arc path is external, the recipient must be considered lucky, and only relatively minor physical injury is expected.

So again, the outcome is crucially dependent on those factors which influence the location of the arc path. It has already been postulated that the likelihood of an internal arc path is high if there is an easy electrical connection to the moist inner parts of the body. If there is no such

connection, and if there are metal electrodes on the surface of the skin, then an external discharge path is more likely, particularly if the surface is moist with perspiration or rain. It is evident that the presence of body orifices close to the entry point of the surge may have a major bearing. Thus, if a person is using a telephone pressed close to the ear and/or mouth, the discharge current will enter the body with severe consequences (electrical breakdown tests have shown that voltages in excess of 10,000 V will normally cause a spark to develop between the telephone and the ear rather than the mouth). If, however, the person is holding the telephone away from the ear, the spark will contact the hand and an external discharge path is more likely. This fortunate result is also likely if the indirect surge occurs when a person is handling an electrical appliance or typing on a computer terminal.

2. Non-Discharge State

There are two situations to consider if the indirect surge voltage is below that needed to cause a discharge arc.

1. The surge voltage is large enough to make a sparking connection to the person (say, greater than 10,000 V), but is below the 200 kV needed for a discharge arc to develop. In this circumstance, (see Figure 3a), the resistance of the body (R_b of between 300 and 1000 Ω, depending on the contact) limits the conductive current to between about 10 to 400 A. The gross physical effects of such currents are likely to be small, because of their relatively small magnitude and because of their short duration (small fractions of a second, as for all lightning stroke currents). Such currents may, of course, impair body sensors and functions which are electrical in nature or are electrically stimulated, particularly if the current passes near or through such sensitive organs as the ear, eye, brain stem, and heart.
2. The surge is too small to make a sparking connection to the body, say, less than the 10,000 V needed to spark between a telephone and an ear. Then no conduction current flows, but as described by Equation 12, a small capacitive current of about 1 A will flow because the voltage is time varying. The effects of this very small and very short-duration current are likely to be small, but electrical stimulation effects cannot be excluded.

C. LIGHTNING INJURIES TO ANIMALS

Medical and observational aspects of lightning injuries to people are detailed in other chapters of this book. Here, a brief description is given of lightning injuries to animals.

Lightning in the field can injure and kill animals by direct strikes and by such indirect effects as touch and step voltage and side flash. The gross electrophysical effects are likely to be similar to those for people. Various research workers have conducted laboratory studies of the effects of electricity and lightning-like surges on animals. A convenient early summary has been provided by Bernstein.[10] In the following discussion, no consideration will be given to the effects of 50- or 60-Hz currents (I_{rms}) or to the influence of duration of exposure.

The best known early analysis of impulse current studies is that of Dalziel,[12] who examined laboratory test data for animals and impulse accident data for people. Dalziel concluded that the hazard from a short-duration electric current (including impulse currents) is related to the energy absorbed, although no attempt was made to link this with a specific physiological explanation. Dalziel has given an energy criterion for the current surges which will give rise to ventricular fibrillation in normal people at the threshold level (1/2% percentile). For a body resistance of about 300 Ω, the threshold energy absorption is about 150 J.

It is generally accepted that larger energy levels are required for bodies of larger mass, e.g., over 1000 J for large farm animals. Kitagawa and colleagues have made more recent and extensive studies of the threshold energies for rabbits and other small animals, and confirmed that the lethal energy is proportional to body mass.[13] The same group of workers used dummies of the human body to study surface flashover effects.[14] The surfaces of the dummies were coated with conductive paint so that the resistance from head to feet was 300 to 500 Ω. It is of interest to note that the recorded stresses for external flashovers were 220 to 270 kV/m and that metal objects influenced the nature of the external flashovers. These matters are similar to surface flashovers of wood. Kitagawa and colleagues also related their studies of surface flashovers on dummies and on small animals to on-the-spot investigations of lightning accidents to people. From these, they concluded that metal objects on the human body tended to enhance the likelihood of external flashover, thus reducing the internal flow of current through the body. Again, the parallel with internal discharges and surface flashovers with wood is clear.

V. MEASUREMENT OF LIGHTNING CURRENTS AND VOLTAGES

If the path of the lightning current is known, straightforward techniques are available to measure the current and voltage. For current measurements, a resistive shunt or a current transformer is inserted in the current path, and the developed voltage is recorded, usually with an oscilloscope. Voltage measurements require the use of a potential divider and oscilloscope. Of course, all the measurement equipment must have a frequency response suited to the rapid variations of voltage and current with time. International standards on high-voltage testing techniques[15] specify the required frequency response. It is sufficient to note here that frequency responses up to at least 10^6 Hz are required to record the microsecond risetimes associated with lightning.

Simpler methods are available for measuring the peak magnitude of the lightning current. The most reliable and widely used methods are the magnetic link or the prerecorded magnetic strip[16] placed near a conductor carrying the lightning current. Both utilize the self-magnetic field of the lightning current. In the former, an initially demagnetized piece of iron is left with a remnant magnetism which can be related directly to the peak current. In the latter, the magnetic field of the lightning current erases part of a signal prerecorded on a piece of magnetic tape. These methods can measure peak lightning currents from 3 to 200 kA with accuracies of about ±5%.

Cruder estimates can be made of the peak lightning current by examining the effects of the current on the materials involved. Lightning currents impinging on or leaving a metal surface cause arc damage craters. Laboratory tests of the effects of lightning currents on various metal surfaces provide information about the crater damage (diameter, discoloration), which can then be used to estimate the peak current. Likewise, lightning currents passing through a porous material such as wood, paper, fiberboard, etc. leave an arc damage hole or furrow. The diameter of the hole or furrow can be related to the peak current, and so provides an estimate of it. Such methods can be used to estimate the peak lightning current with accuracies of about ±25%. If such effects are noted in the investigation of a lightning accident, it may be possible to expose the material involved to artificial lightning currents generated in the laboratory. By testing the material with a range of peak currents, it is possible to "calibrate" the damage effects, and thereby obtain an estimate of the peak magnitude of the real lightning current to within ±10%.

APPENDIX — ELECTRICAL CIRCUITS

Electrical circuits can be analyzed to determine the voltages, currents, and energy absorption associated with the flow of electricity.[1] The circuit components include resistors, inductors, and capacitors, and they constitute an impedance to current flow.

A. RESISTANCE AND RESISTIVE CIRCUITS

The simplest relationship between the voltage (v) across and the current (i) through a component is Ohm's law for resistance (R),

$$v(t) = Ri(t) \tag{1}$$

It is applicable for all values of voltage and current (including time-varying quantities), if R is independent of v and i and is only dependent on the component's physical characteristics — resistivity (ρ), cross-sectional area (A), and length (l); then

$$R = \rho l \,/\, A \tag{2}$$

For nearly all materials, ρ and hence R vary with temperature. For most insulating materials and for resistive materials which pass electricity by ionic conduction, the resistance decreases with increasing temperature (T). Typically, the resistance halves for a 10°C rise in temperature, and the functional relationship between R and T is exponential. The flow of current (I) for a time (t) causes energy (W) to be absorbed in the resistive material, and

$$W = I^2 Rt(J) \tag{3}$$

This energy appears as heat, and so the flow of current may lower the resistance.

There are, of course, many materials which do not conform to Ohm's (linear) law. These are the nonlinear materials, whose resistance is either voltage or current dependent. A common model for nonlinear materials is

$$v = ki^\beta \tag{4}$$

in which k is a material constant (akin to its resistance) and the exponent β describes its degree of nonlinearity. For most of these materials, β is less than 1 and so the v-i characteristics in Figure 2 are typical. (The incremental resistance at any current is the slope of the v-i characteristic.)

Resistors may be connected in series, parallel, or series-parallel combinations to form the circuits required to model electricity flow through a nonhomogeneous object.

If n linear resistors are connected in series, the total resistance R is

$$R = R_1 + R_2 + ... + R_n \tag{5}$$

and, of course, Ohm's law applies for each component and for the combination. In general, the component resistances differ, and while the same current flows through each, their voltages and absorbed energies will differ.

Consider, for example, a voltage of 10,000 V applied for 1 s to three series-connected resistors: $R_1 = 800\,\Omega$, $R_2 = 150\,\Omega$, and $R_3 = 50\,\Omega$. The (common) current is 10 A, and the voltages and absorbed energies are

$$R_1 \quad 8000 \quad V, \quad 80,000 \quad J$$

$$R_2 \quad 1500 \quad V, \quad 15,000 \quad J$$

$$R_3 \quad 500 \quad V, \quad 5,000 \quad J$$

Clearly, most of the voltage and energy absorption is associated with the high-valued resistor R_1, and this may result in major effects on it, e.g., excessive heating or even arcing across it if its electrical breakdown voltage is exceeded.

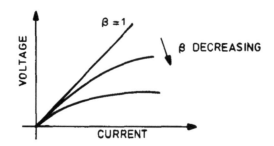

FIGURE 2. Linear and nonlinear voltage-current relationships.

Such a series circuit might model a situation in which electrical connections are made to an object of resistance (R_2) 150 Ω, with one poor contact (R_1) of 800 Ω and a better contact (R_3) of 50 Ω. Clearly, heating or arcing may occur at the entry contact R_1.

If m resistors are connected in parallel, the total resistance is found from

$$1/R = 1/R_2 + 1/R_2 + ... + 1/R_m \tag{6}$$

If the common voltage is V, the total current (I) through the combination is

$$I = V/R \tag{7}$$

and the current (I_i) through each resistor (R_i) is

$$I_i = V/R_i = IR/R_i \tag{8}$$

Clearly, the total current is shared between the component pathways according to the relative magnitudes of their resistances. Consider again 10,000 V applied for 1 s to three resistors connected in parallel: $R_a = 1176.5$ Ω, $R_b = 10,000$ Ω, and $R_c = 20,000$ Ω. The resistance of the parallel combination is 1000 Ω, the total current is 10 A, and the component currents and absorbed energies are:

$$R_a \quad 8.5 \quad A, \quad 85,000 \quad J$$

$$R_b \quad 1 \quad\;\; A, \quad 10,000 \quad J$$

$$R_c \quad 0.5 \quad A, \quad\;\;\; 5000 \quad J$$

Clearly, most of the current flow and energy absorption is associated with the low-valued resistor R_a, and this may cause it to heat excessively.

Consider now what would happen if the three parallel resistors have a negative temperature dependence (i.e., resistance decrease with temperature increase). It is evident that the resistor with the highest energy absorption (R_a) would be the one which would have the highest temperature rise. Therefore, the ratio of its resistance to that of the other two would decrease when compared with the original values, it would therefore carry an even higher proportion of the total current, it would heat up even further, etc. This is an unstable sharing of current between

the three component resistors, and in due course, nearly all the current would flow through the resistance-decreasing and temperature-rising resistor.

This concentration of current into one pathway is characteristic of parallel resistive materials whose resistances decrease with increases in temperature. It can be referred to as runaway thermal breakdown or breakdown by a "decaying" resistor process. The behavior of parallel connected nonlinear resistors is similar. Figure 2 shows that the effective resistance decreases with increasing current, and so leads to current concentration.

B. IMPEDANCE AND CIRCUITS

The modeling of physical objects by electrical circuits often requires the inclusion of inductors and capacitors (as well as resistors). These elements add to the circuit's impedance to current flow, and this impedance (Z) can be described by a generalization of Ohm's law, viz.,

$$v(t) = Z\, i(t) \tag{9}$$

In general, if the electrical quantities are time varying, the voltage and currents have different wave shapes, and hence Z is nonlinear.

As described in Chapter 2, lightning currents and the resulting voltages are time varying, and so it is necessary to consider the contributions of inductance and capacitance. It is sufficient, however, to consider just two combinations: a series-connected resistance and inductance, and a series-connected resistance and capacitance.

The governing equation for a resistance in series with an inductance (L)

$$v(t) = R\, i(t) + L\, di/dt \tag{10}$$

shows that the inductor's contribution to impedance is dependent both on the magnitude of the inductance and on the time rate-of-change of current. For a typical vertical conductor, L is about $1\mu H/m$. A severe lightning current can have a time-to-crest as short as $1\,\mu s$. Consider a lightning current of peak magnitude I passing through an object of length 2 m (L = 2 μH) and resistance R. Substituting into Equation 10,

$$V = RI + 2 \times 10^{-6} \times I / 1 \times 10^{-6}$$

$$V/I = R + 2 \quad (\text{volt}/\text{amp})$$

If R is very small, e.g., <0.1 Ω for a conducting wire, the effective impedance (V/I) is dominated by the inductance. On the other hand, if R is large, e.g., >100 Ω, the inductive contribution is negligible. Some illustrative values can focus the argument. Consider a current of peak value 5000 A with a crest time of 1 μs. If R = 0.1 Ω, V = 10,500 Vp; this is a surprisingly large peak voltage to be developed by a relatively small current across a good conductor (the average current in a direct lightning strike is about 30,000 A). If R = 300 Ω, the prospective voltage developed across the object is 1.5 million V, which is to be expected because of its high resistance (the word prospective has been used because most objects would flash over at a lower voltage).

Insulating materials have a high resistance, and for time-varying electrical quantities, capacitance has a major bearing on current flow. One circuit model is a small resistance in series with a capacitance (C). The relevant equation is

$$v(t) = Ri(t) + (1/C)\int i\, dt \tag{11}$$

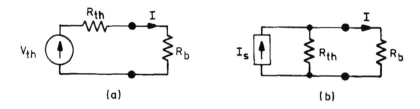

FIGURE 3. Equivalent circuits to determine the current I which flows through an object of resistance R_b.

In the typical circumstance of a voltage surge appearing across an insulating gap (of capacitance C) due to a nearby lightning strike, the main obstacle to the flow of current is the insulator, and so the contribution of normal values of resistance (R) in series is negligible. Then Equation 11 simplifies to

$$v(t) = (1 / C) \int i \, dt$$

and hence

$$i(t) = C \, dv / dt \qquad (12)$$

Consider the capacitance of a small insulating gap between one conductor and another, e.g., a telephone earpiece near a human head, which has a capacitance of about 100 pF. Suppose an incident voltage surge has a magnitude of 10,000 V and a time-to-crest of 1 μs. From Equation 12, I = 1 A, and this capacitive current will flow through the circuit even if the resistance of the insulating gap is infinite. (Note that the effective impedance is large (10,000 Ω) compared with the magnitude of any series-connected resistance.) Capacitive current will only flow while the voltage is changing with time.

C. THE THÉVENIN EQUIVALENT CIRCUIT

In a lightning strike event, the consequences of damage and injury are very dependent on the current flow through the stricken object. Thévenin's theorem provides a simple procedure for determining this current for a wide range of circumstances.

Let the object have a resistance R_b between the entry and exit points of current flow. Then, when a lightning strike occurs to or near to the object, the physical system which delivers the current to it can be described by either of the two equivalent circuits given in Figure 3.

In Figure 3a, V_{th} is the open-circuit voltage which would appear if the stricken object was not connected, while in Figure 3b, I_s is the current which would flow if the object was short-circuited (i.e., R_b set to zero). The Thévenin voltage V_{th} and the short-circuit current I_s are related by $R_{th} = V_{th}/I_s$.

Once the equivalent circuit has been determined, it is straightforward to calculate the current I which will flow through a stricken object of resistance R_b; quite simply,

$$I = V_{th} / (R_{th} + R_b) \qquad (13)$$

REFERENCES

1. **Skilling, H. H.,** *Electrical Engineering Circuits,* John Wiley & Sons, 1965 (or any textbook on electrical circuits).

2. **Darveniza, M., et al.,** Modelling for Lightning Performance Calculations, *IEEE Trans. Power Appar. Syst.,* 98, 1900, 1979.

3. **Stringfellow, M. F.,** Lightning induced overvoltages on overhead distribution lines, *IEE Conf Publ. (London),* 236, 26, 1984.

4. **Power, S., Darveniza, M., and Mackerras, D.,** Lightning protection — an analytical approach to protection design, in Proc. Conf. Inst. Eng., Australia, Darwin, 1987, 271.

5. **Uman, M. A.,** *Understanding Lightning,* Bek, Carnegie, PA, 1971; reissued as *All About Lightning,* Dover, New York, 1986.

6. **Darveniza, M.,** *The Electrical Properties of Wood and Line Design,* University of Queensland Press, Brisbane, 1980.

7. **Wallis, N. K.,** *The Australian Timber Handbook,* Angus and Robertson, Sydney, 1970.

8. **Defandorf, F. M.,** Electrical resistance to earth of a live tree, *Trans. AIEE.,* 75(3), 936, 1956.

9. **Ganong, W. S.,** *Review of Medical Physiology,* Lange, Los Altos, CA, 1983.

10. **Bernstein, T.,** Effects of electricity and lightning on man and animals, *J. Forsenic Sci.,* 18, 3, 1973.

11. **Dalziel, C. F.,** Re-evaluation of lethal electric currents, *IEEE Trans. Ind. Gen. Appl.,* 4, 467, 1968.

12. **Dalziel, C. F.,** A study of the hazards of impulse currents, *Trans. Am. Inst. Electr. Eng. Part 3,* 72, 1032, 1953.

13. **Ishikawa, T., Ohashi, M., Kitagawa, N., et al.,** Experimental study on the lethal threshold value of multiple successive voltage impulses to rabbits simulating multi-stroke lightning flash, *Int. J. Biometeor.,* 29, 157, 1986.

14. **Kitagawa, N., Turumi, S., Ishikawa, T., and Ohashi, M.,** The nature of lightning discharges on human bodies and the basis for safety and protection, in Proc. 18th. Int. Conf. Lightning Protection, Munich, 1985, 435.

15. Standards Association of Australia, *High Voltage Testing Techniques, A.S. 1931-1976* (and similar national standards based on I.E.C. Publ. 60).

16. **Darveniza, M.,** The measurement of impulse current using a pre-magnetised tape, *J.E.E.E.A. Inst. Eng. Aust. IREE Aust.,* 6, 74, 1986.

Chapter 4

OCCURRENCE OF LIGHTNING DEATH AND INJURY

David Mackerras

TABLE OF CONTENTS

I. INTRODUCTION

The information presented in this chapter is based on reports and papers relating to lightning-caused death and injury for the U.S., England and Wales, Singapore, and Australia. For the U.S., basic information on fatalities and injuries is presented in *Storm Data*.[1] Bernstein[2] and Zegel[3] have used these and other data as the bases for their analyses. Golde and Lee[4] have presented statistics for England and Wales, Chao et al.[5] analyzed 80 deaths for the period 1956 to 1979 for Singapore, and Prentice[6] has analyzed 286 lightning-caused deaths in Australia for the period 1920 to 1969.

The authors have commented on various uncertainties in the data; perhaps the major problem is that of lightning-caused deaths or injuries that are not included in the analysis for some reason. From a worldwide viewpoint, there are many countries with large populations for which no reports or papers were available; thus, the available data should be viewed as an imperfect sample from which some deductions about worldwide lightning-caused death and injury rates can be made. There is a large uncertainty in these deductions.

II. HISTORICAL TRENDS IN LIGHTNING-CAUSED DEATH AND INJURY RATES

Lightning-caused death rates are usually expressed as the number of deaths per million of population per year. For a given country, this death rate usually exhibits significant year to year fluctuations, so averaging over a 5- or 10-year period is appropriate to smooth out short-term fluctuations. Figure 1 presents the available data of this type for the period 1920 to 1980, for the U.S., England and Wales, Singapore, and Australia, with single average values for South Africa, Austria, and West Germany also shown.

The data for the U.S. for 1922 to 1967 were obtained from Golde and Lee,[4] and data for the period 1959 to 1983 were derived from *Storm Data*.[1] Five-year averages were used for each of these data sets. There is a significant discrepancy between the two data sets in the overlap period 1961 to 1967. In deriving the death rates for 1959 to 1983, the population of the U.S. was assumed to be 200×10^6 in 1969, and to increase linearly at a rate of 2.5×10^6 per year.

The most notable historical trend apparent from Figure 1 is a general downward trend in death rates from relatively high values in the decade 1930 to 1940 to lower values in the decade 1970 to 1980. This has been attributed to increasing urbanization of population, and possibly to a more widespread public awareness of the risk of lightning injury and death, and appropriate steps to avoid danger. The downward trend may also be associated with a long-term decrease in thunderstorm activity. In Brisbane, Australia, Mackerras[7] reported a drop in the 10-year average thunderdays per year from about 43 in 1930 to about 24 in 1968. Changnon[8] reported that thunderstorm day frequencies in the central and eastern U.S., Japan, South Africa, and parts of southern Europe were 10 to 30% below their 70-year averages during the period 1951 to 1970.

III. LIGHTNING-CAUSED INJURY RATES

Comparable lightning-caused injury and death rates are given in *Storm Data*[1] and by Zegel.[3]

For the period 1959 to 1985, for the U.S., there were 2566 deaths and 6720 injuries,[1] excluding 81 people killed in an aircraft crash on December 8, 1963, attributed to lightning. This gives a ratio of injuries to deaths of about 2.6. Zegel[3] reported 960 killed and 1736 injured for the period 1959 to 1965 inclusive, giving a ratio of about 1.8. Using this ratio, one can infer the number of persons injured, given the number of persons killed.

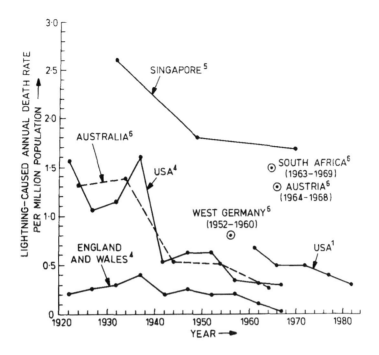

FIGURE 1. Lightning-caused annual death rate per million of population plotted against time. Five-year averages are shown for the U.S., England, and Wales; 10-year averages are shown for Australia. (From References 1, 4, 5, and 6.)

IV. DISTRIBUTION OF LIGHTNING-CAUSED DEATH RATE BY SEX

All sources indicate that male deaths exceed female deaths by a large factor. Zegel[3] reported for the U.S. that 75 to 85% (mean 80%) of lightning fatalities are male and 15 to 25% (mean 20%) are female. Chao et al.[5] reported 66 male and 14 female deaths for Singapore over the 24-year period 1956 to 1979. Prentice[6] reported 252 male and 34 female deaths in Australia in the 50-year period 1920 to 1969. We define the factor k_s as the ratio of the fraction of deaths for the particular sex divided by the fraction of the population of that sex, assumed to be 0.5. Table 1 summarizes the above data in terms of k_s values.

Thus, the male death rate is about 1.67 times the whole-population average death rate, and the female death rate is about 0.33 times the whole-population average death rate.

V. DISTRIBUTION OF LIGHTNING-CAUSED DEATH RATE BY AGE

Distributions of lightning-caused deaths by age have been provided by Prentice[6] for Australia over the 25-year period 1945 to 1969, and by Chao et al.[5] for Singapore over the 24-year period 1956 to 1979. Their observations are summarized in Table 2.

The quantity k_a is defined as the ratio of the fraction of all lightning-caused deaths in a given age group to the fraction of the population in that age group.

Values of k_a are plotted in Figure 2 against age for 10-year age groups, for Australia and Singapore. This shows that the highest risk group consists of 20 to 29-year-old persons, with a

TABLE 1
Distribution of Lightning-Caused Death by Sex

Country	Item	Male	Female	Ref.
U.S.	Fractions of deaths	0.8	0.2	3
	k_s values	1.6	0.4	
Singapore	Fraction of deaths	0.825	0.175	5
	k_s values	1.65	0.35	
Australia	Fraction of deaths	0.88	0.12	6
	k_s values	1.76	0.24	
	Mean k_s values	1.67	0.33	

TABLE 2
Distribution of Lightning-Caused Death by Age

Country (period)	Age range (years)	Number of deaths in age group	Fraction of deaths in age group	Fraction of population in age group	k_a	Ref.
Australia	0—9	4	0.0396	0.207	0.191	6
(1945—1969)	10—19	23	0.2277	0.157	1.450	
	20—29	30	0.2970	0.135	2.200	
	30—39	14	0.1386	0.149	0.930	
	40—49	7	0.0693	0.131	0.529	
	50—59	14	0.1386	0.098	1.414	
	60—69	9	0.0891	0.073	1.221	
	70+	0	0	0.050	0	
Singapore	0—9	7	0.0875	0.295	0.297	5
(1956—1979)	10—19	25	0.3125	0.245	1.276	
	20—29	21	0.2625	0.139	1.888	
	30—39	12	0.150	0.118	1.271	
	40—49	13	0.1625	0.086	1.890	
	50—59	1	0.0125	0.067	0.187	
	60—69	1	0.0125	0.036	0.347	

risk of lightning-caused death about twice that of the whole population. Both curves show a second peak at the 40 to 49-year-old group for Singapore and the 50 to 59-year-old group for Australia.

The estimated lightning death rate for a particular age group may be obtained by multiplying the mean whole-population death rate by k_a.

VI. TYPES OF LOCATIONS AND ACTIVITIES OF PERSONS WHEN KILLED BY LIGHTNING

Zegel[3] has provided information on the type of location and activity of some of the persons killed or injured by lightning on the continental U.S. for the 7-year period 1959 to 1965 inclusive, as shown in Table 3. Percentages are based on a total of 960 persons killed by lightning in the sample period.

Prentice[6] has provided information on the type of location and activity of persons killed by lightning, divided into two 13-year periods, 1945 to 1957 and 1957 to 1969, for Australia. His observations are summarized in Table 4.

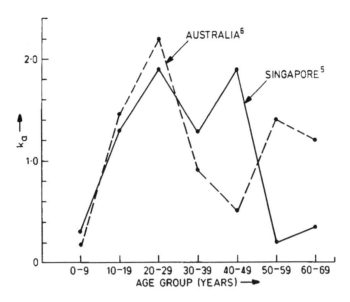

FIGURE 2. The factor k_a plotted against age group for Singapore (Reference 5) and Australia (Reference 6). The factor k_a is the ratio of the fraction of lightning-caused deaths for that age group to the fraction of the population in that age group.

TABLE 3
Location and Activity of Persons Killed by Lightning[3]

Type of location or activity	Number of persons killed	Number of persons injured	Percentage of total killed
Under trees	102	120	10.6
Open water	78	70	8.1
Tractors	69	60	7.2
Golf	36	68	3.8
Telephone	4	36	0.4

The information in Table 4 shows that lightning deaths predominantly occur outdoors; indoor deaths are usually associated with small sheds, often with low metal roofs and no conducting path to ground, such as a milking shed. The table also shows that the proportion of deaths associated with recreation is increasing with time, a trend also note by Chao et al.[5] for Singapore.

VII. SEASONAL AND DIURNAL VARIATION IN THE OCCURRENCE OF LIGHTNING-CAUSED DEATHS

The seasonal variation in the occurrence of lightning-caused deaths has been reported by Prentice[6] for Australia, by Chao et al.[5] for Singapore, and in *Storm Data*[1] for the U.S. From this information, the cumulative percentages of lightning-caused deaths has been calculated and plotted in Figure 3. For convenience in comparing these curves, the 12-month period begins in July for the Southern Hemisphere (Figure 3a) and in January for the Northern Hemisphere (Figure 3b).

The similarity in the curves for Australia and the U.S. should be noted, allowing for the 6-month shift between the two curves. The curves show that the majority (about 80%) of all deaths occur between October and February inclusive in Australia. In the U.S., about 80% of deaths occur between June and September inclusive.

In Figure 3a, the cumulative percentage of lightning occurrence over the 12-month period is

TABLE 4
Persons Killed by Lightning Outdoors and Indoors, at Work and Recreation[6]

Type of location and activity	1945–1957		1957–1969	
	Number killed	%	Number killed	%
Outdoors, at work	40	66.7 } 95	17	44.7 } 94.7
Outdoors, recreation	17	28.3	19	50
Indoors, at work	2	3.3 } 5	2	5.3 } 5.3
Indoors, recreation	1	1.7	0	0
Total	60		38	

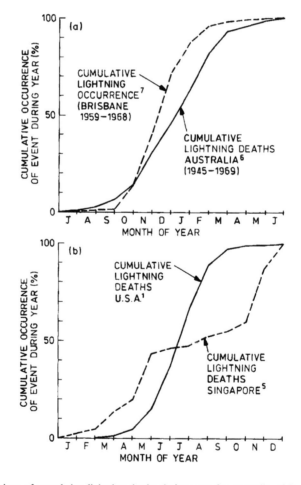

FIGURE 3. Comparison of cumulative lightning deaths during year for Australia, U.S., and Singapore, with cumulative lightning occurrence for Australia. (From References 1, 5, 6, and 7.)

also shown. This curve was derived from data in Mackerras[7] and is based on lightning observations in Brisbane between 1959 and 1968. Lightning activity in Brisbane is fairly typical of that over much of the eastern states of Australia where the majority of deaths were recorded.

TABLE 5
Diurnal Variation in Occurrence of Lightning-Caused
Deaths. Percentages of Deaths in Time Intervals Shown

Local Time (h)	U.S. 1959–1965[a]	Australia 1945–1969[b]
0000		
	1% }	11%
0060		
	10%	
1200		
		9% }
1400	70%	43% } 85%
1600		33%
1800		
		4% }
2000	20%	} 4%
		0%
2400		

[a] From Zegel, F. H., *Weatherwise*, 20(4), 169, 1967.
[b] From Prentice, S. A., *Electr. Eng. Trans. Inst. Eng. Aust.*, EE8(2), 55, 1972.

The similarity in the two curves indicates that the rate of occurrence of lightning deaths is approximately proportional to the rate of occurrence of lightning flashes to ground.

Information on the diurnal variation in lightning-caused deaths has been provided by Prentice[6] and Zegel.[3] Their data are summarized in Table 5.

These data clearly show that the period 1200 to 1800 hours local time is the most dangerous, with the majority of deaths, 70% for the U.S. and 85% for Australia. The period coincides with the maximum rate of occurrence of lightning, and is also mainly within normal work and outdoor recreation hours.

VIII. INFERRED WORLDWIDE LIGHTNING DEATH RATE

On the basis of information from countries with approximately known lightning death rates, the rate can be estimated from the thunderday level. Using the information summarized in Figure 1 as a guide, the approximate death rates are shown in Table 6.

Assuming a mean annual worldwide rate of 0.3 per 10^6 population, and taking the 1970 world population at 3.6×10^9, an annual worldwide death rate at that time of about 1000 can be inferred.

In order to assess the probability that a ground flash will kill a person, we may estimate the number of ground flashes per year as follows. As stated in Chapter 2, there are about 100 flashes per second worldwide. About 20% of these are ground flashes. Thus, the number of ground flashes per year is 20 times the number of seconds per year, or about 6×10^8. Thus, about one ground flash in 6×10^5 kills a person.

As a check on this estimate, the information in Figure 2 of Prentice[6] was used, showing that in an area of about 1.8×10^6 km^2 covering the main population centers in the eastern states of Australia, there were about 60 deaths in 25 years. Assuming that the ground flash density for Brisbane, 1.2 km^{-2} year^{-1}, is an average for the whole region, there were $1.8 \times 10^6 \times 1.2 \times 25 = 5 \times 10^7$ ground flashes in the 25-year period. Thus, about one ground flash in 8×10^5 caused death, in reasonable agreement with the figure obtained from the worldwide inferred death rate. In the area under consideration, the thunderday level ranges from about 10 to 50 per year.

TABLE 6
Thunderdays per Year and Lightning-Caused Death Rate

Typical range in thunderdays per year	Approximate mean annual lightning death rate per 10^6 population
5—20	0.2
20—40	0.4
40—80	1.0
80—200	1.7

IX. CONCLUSION

Lightning-caused, long-term mean annual death rates in various countries range from about 0.2 to 1.7 per million of population, corresponding to a range of annual thunderday levels from about 10 in higher altitudes to over 100 in tropical climates. There are anecdotal reports of considerably higher lightning death rates among some African populations. There has been a slow decline in annual death rates since the 1930s in England and Wales, the U.S., Singapore, and Australia. The proportion of persons killed during recreation has been rising, while the proportion of persons killed at work has been falling. The available information makes it plausible that the lightning death rate is directly related to the rate of occurrence of ground flashes. Thus, the seasonal variation of death rate follows closely the seasonal variation of lightning occurrence, both having their highest values in the local summer months. Similarly, the diurnal variation in lightning death rates follows closely the diurnal variation in lightning occurrence, both having their highest values in the 1200 to 1800 hours local time period. The number of persons injured by lightning is about 2.5 times the number killed.

The lightning death rate for males is about 1.67 times the whole-population average and the death rate for females is about 0.33 times the whole-population average. The 20- to 29-year-old age group has about twice the death rate of the whole population. The group at greatest risk is males aged 20 to 29 years, whose death rate is about 3.3 times the whole-population average.

Estimates of the probability that a ground flash will kill a person were made by two methods. From one method, it is estimated that one ground flash in 6×10^5 causes death. From the other method, one ground flash in 8×10^5 causes death. An estimate of the annual lightning-caused death rate for a particular location can be made using the annual thunderday level as shown in Table 6.

REFERENCES

1. National Oceanic and Atmospheric Administration, *Storm Data*, 27(12), 1985.
2. **Bernstein, T.,** *Lightning Death and Injury in the United States, Fourteen Years (1968—1981)*, Department of Electrical and Computer Engineering, University of Wisconsin, Madison, 1982.
3. **Zegel, F. H.,** Lightning deaths in the United States: a seven-year survey from 1959 to 1965, *Weatherwise*, 20(4), 169, 1967.
4. **Golde, R. H. and Lee, W. R.,** Death by Lightning, *Proc. Inst. Electr. Eng.*, 123(10R), 1163, 1976.
5. **Chao, T. C., Pakiam, J. E., and Chia, J.,** A study of lightning deaths in Singapore, *Singapore Med. J.*, 22(3), 150, 1981.
6. **Prentice, S. A.,** Lightning fatalities in Australia, *Electr. Eng. Trans. Inst. Eng. Aust.*, 8(2), 55, 1972.
7. **Mackerras, D.,** Prediction of lightning incidence and effects in electrical systems, *Electr. Eng. Trans. Inst. Eng. Aust.*, 14(2), 73, 1978.
8. **Changnon, S. A.,** Secular trends in thunderstorm frequency, in *Electrical Processes in Atmospheres*, Dolezalek, H. and Reiter, R., Eds., Steinkopff, Darmstadt, 1977, 482.

Chapter 5

CLINICAL PRESENTATION OF THE LIGHTNING VICTIM

C. J. Andrews and M. A. Cooper
(with a contribution by M. J. Eadie)

TABLE OF CONTENTS

I. INTRODUCTION

As in all branches of medical practice, the injunction to "take a history and examine the patient" as the cardinal approach to diagnosis is entirely applicable to those who are injured by lightning. It is only in the proper eliciting and interpretation of symptoms and signs that proper diagnosis is made, and on which appropriate treatment is based.

If possible, it is helpful to get a history from bystanders as to what happened. Unfortunately, probably because a lightning incident happens so quickly, there are frequently as many versions as there are bystanders. However, while the history should not stop the physician from doing a complete evaluation if certain historical information is missing, it can often be useful in explaining some of the injuries found.

It is also important to the patient's care to determine if there are any other matters which should concern the physician such as allergies, medications, and concurrent illnesses, particularly heart and lung problems and diabetes. Sometimes the patient will be alert enough to give this information. More often, however, the patient is unconscious or confused at initial presentation, so that this information must be obtained from others.

This chapter, therefore, addresses the constellation of symptoms and signs that may be seen in the lightning-injured patient. Initially, a survey will place the features in perspective, and this will be followed by a systematic examination of symptoms and signs. This leads to a short discussion of differential diagnosis, and it will be seen that this is of forensic significance. The pronouncement of death in the lightning injured concludes this chapter.

Chapter 6 will present the pathophysiology — the theoretical basis — of these injuries. Chapter 7 will discuss the care of lightning-injured patients and the priorities in their evaluation. No attempt is therefore made to address genesis of the symptoms and signs at this stage. This topic is dealt with in Chapter 6.

II. A NUMERICAL AND CASE-STUDY PERSPECTIVE

A. A NUMERICAL PERSPECTIVE

Lightning injury can produce an enormous spectrum of clinical symptoms and signs ranging from the common (e.g., cardiac asystole, respiratory arrest, keraunoparalysis, arborescent markings, etc.) to the rare (e.g., disseminated intravascular coagulation, intracerebral hemorrhage, etc.). To enable the relative frequency of symptoms and signs to be gauged, a collation of literature reports since 1900 has been undertaken, and the relative frequency of reported features is shown in Table 1. This tabulation is to be compared with an earlier one by Cooper.[64] In that review, 205 cases from the literature were considered, of which 66 were analyzed. These cases have all been included in the current survey except those dealing with lightning accidents in pregnancy, which was considered too specialized for the current purpose.

The present tabulation drew 221 cases from 58 papers published up to 1987. Cases were selected from those found in the literature which were judged to be reported in adequate detail for the appraisal of a relatively full clinical history. Thus, several cases are not included on the basis of the present authors' subjective judgment of their detail.

The constellation of symptoms reported in Table 1 is summarized under the headings of neurologic, cardiac, ocular, otic, gastrointestinal, pulmonary, musculoskeletal, traumatic, hematological, and external injuries. The total number of each injury is found, and the percentage of the total sample exhibiting this injury is tabulated. For purposes of comparison, those figures obtained from Cooper[64] are also shown for the symptoms she considered.

The total number of cases differs slightly for some symptoms since some authors (e.g., Reference 76) give exact figures for some symptoms, while reporting "many" or "few" suffering from others. Only exact numbers have been used.

TABLE 1
Relative Frequency of Findings

Symptom/sign	No.	Cases	% of cases (see note)		Symptom/sign	No.	Cases	% of cases (see note)	
Neurological									
Loss of conc.	130	221	59	(72)	Cranial nerve abn.	11	221	5	
Restlessness	26	221	12		Peripheral nerve abnormality	6	221	3	
Depression	7	221	3		Hyperthermia	10	221	5	
Weakness	8	186	4		Hypothermia	4	221	2	
Para/ hypoesthesia	37	221	17		Low. extrem. paral.	77	186	41	(69)
Cerebral edema	6	221	3		Upp. extrem. paral.	54	186	29	(30)
Intracranial bleeding	5	221	2		Amnesia	86	186	46	(86)
Pyramidal signs	4	221	2		Convulsions	6	221	3	
Hyporeflexia	7	221	4		Fract. skull	6	221	3	
Cardiac									
Arrest	45	221	20	(30)	Tachycardia	21	221	10	
"Shock"	19	221	9		T-wave change	17	221	8	
Hypertension	8	221	4		ST change	22	221	10	
Bradycardia	7	221	3						
Ocular									
Photophobia	2	221	1		Corneal opacity	3	221	1	
Cataract	7	221	3		Macular abnormal.	4	221	2	
Retinal edema	3	221	1		Visual loss	13	221	6	
Otic									
Ruptured eardrum	21	221	10	(50)	Otorrhea	4	221	2	
Deafness	16	221	7						
GI abnormality	7	221	3						
Pulmonary									
Pneumonia	5	221	2		Pulm. Contusion/ edema	5	221	2	
Tachypnea	5	221	2						
Musculoskeletal/Renal/Hematological									
Hematuria/ myoglobinuria	10	221	5		Marjolin ulcer	1	221	1	
DIC	1	221	1						
External									
Burns, head	59	186	32	(44)	Burns, leg	68	186	37	(55)
Burns, trunk	85	186	46	(66)	No burns	27	221	12	(11)
Burns, arm	42	186	23	(30)					
Other									
Clothing damage	11	221	5		Mortality	43	221	20	(30)

Note: Figures from Cooper[64] in parentheses where applicable.

From Andrews, C. J. and Darveniza, M., *Adv. Trauma*, 4, 241, 1989. With permission.

In general, it may be seen that some symptoms are well represented and others appear only rarely. Among the common symptoms are loss of consciousness (59%), restlessness, hysteria, or dizziness (12%), presence of paresthesia or hypoesthesia (17%), presence of keraunoparalysis (41%), upper limb paralysis (29%), and amnesia (46%). In the cardiovascular system, cardiopulmonary arrest occurred in 20% of the cases, and electrocardiographic abnormalities in approximately 10% of cases. Surprisingly, ocular symptoms were only rarely reported, compared with an incidence of 55% sustaining some ocular injury quoted by Smith.[75] This is attributed to the specialized nature of the injuries, which may pass unnoticed in general reports. The remaining commonly occurring injuries were burns, which, depending on the site, occurred at rates of 23 and 46%.

Among the minor symptoms reported, some are surprising by their relatively low level of occurrence. Cerebral edema, hyperflexia, hyporeflexia, hyperthermia, hypertension, bradycardia, ruptured tympanic membrane, and damage to clothing would all seem to be underestimated from the qualitative impression one gains from reading the literature.

Cooper's previous figures may be compared with those of this survey. In general, in each of Cooper's categories a higher incidence of a particular symptom was found. The trends of the current percentages, however, closely follow those in her report. Overall, the mortality recorded in this survey was 20%, compared with 30% recorded by Cooper.

In any review of this nature, certain biases are inevitable, and they affect the representativeness of the injury proportion obtained. The biases include the following. Not all cases of lightning strike are reported in the literature. Those of a more minor nature are not published. There is thus an underestimate of minor injuries found by this method. This bias has been quantified,[64] giving an injury rate that is four to five times more than that reported by accounts detailing case fatalities. Further, only serious cases are generally considered to have sufficient interest to publish in the literature. Thus, serious injuries tend to be overestimated in a survey by this method. In the presentation of cases, symptoms are selectively reported by different authors to suit the purpose of their given paper. This does not imply any malintent. For example, it is reasonable that a paper on the ocular complications of lightning strike should not report in detail the gastrointestinal findings of an injured person. Again, this may lead to a loss of relativity of some symptoms.

B. A CASE-STUDY PERSPECTIVE

Accounts of cases detail varying severity. The following are included verbatim, and will provide the reader with a feeling for the type of history to be expected:

From Apfelberg et al.:[20]

Case 1. J.R., a 9 year old girl, was struck by lightning while standing on a large metal playground slide. Observers stated that the bolt struck the child directly in the chest and that she "lit up." This was followed by a convulsion and unconsciousness lasting about 10 to 15 min.

On admission 45 min after injury, the patient was restless, hysterical, and semi-comatose, with a blood pressure of 104/70 mm Hg and a pulse of 140. Second-degree burns were present over the anterior abdomen and thighs, with no evidence of entrance or exit burns. Both feet were cold, mottled, and cyanotic, with no palpable pulses below the femoral arteries at the groin and with minimal sensation.

The patient was resuscitated with a Ringer's lactate infusion, and was given oxygen, digitalis, and aminophylline for pulmonary edema. Fasciotomies of the lower extremities were considered, but were not performed because gradual improvement in both color and sensation occurred over the next several hours. During the first 8 h,

low molecular weight dextran (Rheomacrodex) was given to improve the microcirculation of the lower extremities. Urine hemoglobin and myoglobin were 3+ for 48 hr, then returned to normal. All laboratory and clinical parameters were normal by 4 days following trauma, and the patient was discharged on the sixth post-injury day. Subsequent follow-up reveals no residual deformity.

From Ravitch et al.[1] (edited by the present author):

Shortly before 3:30 p.m. on the afternoon of July 24, 1959, a 10 year old boy started to cycle home from a motion picture showing at a school in Baltimore County, to avoid impending rain. He was followed soon after by 2 children who saw the lightning strike "just in front of us" and found the boy slumped over his bicycle against a tree, unconscious. The intervals were established by a check with the tape of the local fire station, which received the ambulance call at 3:28 p.m., and by retracing and timing of the movements of the children. One of them cycled back to the school, summoned help, returned to the victim and then cycled to a telephone to put in the call. Not less than 5 minutes elapsed before the ambulance call. The patient was carried to the school, thought by a boy scout to have a palpable pulse and given back-pressure, arm-lift artificial respiration by the scout.

The ambulance arrived at 3:32, when attempts at use of an automatic cycling respirator failed, and the victim was rushed to the hospital at 3:38 p.m. The boy scout found the pulse still present at this point. During transportation, attempts at ventilation with the resuscitator again failed. The ambulance arrived at the Baltimore City Hospital at 3:45 p.m.; the body had not been seen to breathe at any time, and the artificial respiration had ceased some time before 3:38 p.m.

When he was brought into the accident room he was apparently dead. The face was deathly pale, the lips slightly cyanotic and the pupils widely dilated. He was pulseless and did not breathe. At 3:46 mouth-to-airway breathing was instituted, with a double-ended oropharyngeal airway, and the left side of the chest was opened anteriorly. The chest wall did not bleed. The heart was motionless, not dilated and not fibrillating. Massage of the heart was begun, and after 1 or 2 minutes, 2 ml. of a 1:1000 solution of epinephrine was injected into the left ventricle, time not being taken to prepare the preferable 1:10,000 solution. With 1 or 2 more compressions of the heart vigorous contractions resumed at 3:50 p.m. The systolic pressure was recorded at 110 almost at once. At 3:55 p.m., with the chest still open, the patient was packed in crushed ice and the oropharyngeal airway replaced by an intratracheal tube for manual bag-pressure respiration. The pupils, dilated when he was first seen, narrowed by 4:05 p.m. but did not react to light. Intravenous infusions of fluids had been administered from the outset. No anesthesia was required for the thoracotomy closure. He was making ineffective respiratory movements, and the pupils now reacted to light. On the operating table and thereafter hypothermia was continued with a cooling mattress. A tracheostomy was performed and a Foley catheter was inserted into the bladder.

• • • •

In the late afternoon of the 3rd day the boy's father thought that he had opened his eyes when his name was called. There were no further convulsions, but the patient, so far as the staff had observed, was comatose all day. Late in the evening he moved all the extremities at times, effective spontaneous respirations were resumed, and the respirator was used only intermittently for the next 36 hours.

• • • •

On the 16th day he first asked for food and managed to sit up. By August 10, the 18th day, neurologic examination showed minimal cerebellar signs and persistent but mild signs of hemiplegia.

Recovery was progressive, and he was discharged from the hospital on August 22, 1959, 29 days after the injury. There were no evidences of emotional or personality changes. There was a moderate tremor of the hands, which was perhaps due to weakness, and a peculiar nasal quality to the voice. He returned to school and was considered unchanged in behavior and ability. His I.Q. was just a little higher than when it had been determined before his accident indicating no measurable change in this response to formal testing.

He now performs at his previous level in school and is active in games and bicycling.

Personal communication to one author (C.J.A.):

It happened during the course of an annual Bowling Club Picnic on the shoreline of our beautiful Lake Macquarie—quite a large expanse of water. The picnic was held in a very large park on the water's edge. I was there with 5 of my children. Our family has attended the picnic for possibly the last 15 years with only the last three being held in this park (Speers Point Park). This year my husband was away in Sydney for a State Trial Bowls game and my 18-year-old son drove us there, a journey of about 15 minutes from home. When we arrived at the park a little later than usual we noticed that there were more people in the park than usual. I later learned that there was a Swimming Carnival taking place in the pool across the road.

As usual we sat under a tree with our belongings, as sunburn can be a problem in hot weather. There was one tree available next to the jetty and it was a very large tree. We had been there about an hour with the storm clouds gathered. My 18-year-old son and 16-year-old daughter went to the shop by car — about 5 minutes away. Not long after they left the wind started to blow in strong gusts. Two of my children had entered the water for a swim. As the storm was beginning I told my youngest child, who had remained with me, to tell the swimmers to come out of the water. Just then a T-shirt blew away and I went to retrieve it. The folding chair I was sitting on blew over and I placed the chair on top of the T-shirt and went to sit on the stumpy part of the tree at the base. It was uncomfortable to sit on so I put a couple of towels over it and sat down. My daughter had returned telling me that the swimmers were coming out of the water. She was standing about 5 feet away. I picked up an umbrella (a wooden one from Singapore) as it was now starting to rain and becoming very windy. As I went to open the umbrella there was a bang and a white flash (I felt as if the umbrella had exploded) then a feeling of being flung. Next was a searing burning feeling in the area where I had been sitting. Someone spoke to me. I later found out it was my daughter who had been swimming. I told her that I didn't know what was happening to me. At that stage I was lying face down and stretched out on the ground. I was screaming. Then a lady came to me and told me I was all right and I felt calmer. I was having some difficulty in breathing.

A young man drove his blue van over to where I was lying. By now it was raining very heavily. Four men lifted me into the back of the van. Some people talked to me until the ambulance arrived. The police were also there. We drove slowly to the Wallsend Hospital. Both my legs were numb but gradually the feeling came back an hour later. Halfway there the burns began stinging very badly and I was given an oxygen mask. At the hospital I was given morphine and tetanus injections. I was taken to the Acute Surgical Unit and hospitalized for 2 days. Burns were dressed on a four-hourly basis.

Some comments from people who were in the park at the time of the strike: The noise was described as deafening. A photo of the tree indicated the damage about 100 feet up. I heard that people dropped things they were carrying and dropped to the ground. My youngest daughter who was near me when it happened fell over and had three tears in her sandshoe she was wearing. Other articles of clothing under the tree were damaged with either tears or burn marks. My 16-year-old daughter told me that the towels I was sitting on were stuck to my dress and that they suddenly fell off my dress.

These cases provide a "feeling" for the commonly reported experience of lightning injury. We now turn to documenting the symptomatology.

In setting out the injuries presenting due to lightning injury, one particular point needs strong emphasis. Lightning injury, though electrical in nature, is quite a different phenomenon from injury due to "technical" electricity. The differences in etiology and presentation are summarized in Table 2. From this follows the important maxim that the treatment of these two injuries differs markedly. This will be elaborated in later chapters.

A further means of comparing findings in lightning injury is the collation of post-mortem examination reports. In Queensland, Australia, a formal index of causes of death from archived reports dates from 1935. All reports since that date have been examined by the author and the findings collated to form Table 3. In each case, the patient was found dead after the injury and came to the coroner's attention in this way.

We now present symptoms and signs of lightning injury considered by bodily system. One thing will become apparent as we proceed, and that is the variability of presentations seen.

III. CARDIORESPIRATORY SYSTEMS

A. CARDIOVASCULAR SYSTEM

The most serious presentation seen is that of the patient in cardiorespiratory arrest, and this is classically said to be asystolic arrest.[1,2] This is, of course, an emergency and requires urgent management.

Other arrhythmias have also been documented. Commonly accepted dogma[2] is that the heart, after standstill, restarts in sinus bradycardia, but is overcome once more by a secondary hypoxic arrest due to pulmonary standstill. Andrews et al.[62] have reported experiments suggesting the sequence to be initial asystole followed by a small period of bradycardia, then intense tachycardia leading to secondary hypoxic arrest.

Ventricular premature contractions may be seen,[28] as may sinus pauses with escape.[9] Atrial fibrillation has been reported[3] which reverted after treatment within 24 h. Ventricular fibrillation has been more recently reported,[11-14] and may be more common than is classically stated.[11] Ventricular tachycardia during treatment has been seen.[28]

Electrocardiographic signs are widespread and variable, and have been used to support various arguments over the pathogenesis of the findings. Most ECG signs resolve completely, but may take up to 12 months to do so.

Sinha[4] classifies ECG findings into three groups:

1. Myocardial injury — infarction type
2. Myocardial injury — ischemic type
3. Cardiac standstill of initial presentation

Various, and all, patterns of infarction changes may be seen. Sinha[4] reports T-wave inversions in leads II, III, aVF, V_3, and V_4 immediately after injury. These deepened subsequently and spread to include V_2 and V_5. ST elevation subsequently appeared in V_2 and V_3, and a Q-wave in aVL. Chest pain was consistent with infarction. Resolution with only nonspecific T-wave changes persisting at 2 months occurred (see Figure 1).

TABLE 2

Comparison Between Lightning Injury and That from "Technical" Electricity

Factor	Lightning	High voltage
Time of exposure	Brief and impulsive	Prolonged
Peak current range	3,000–200,000 Amperes	10–10,000 Amperes
Type of current	Undirectional	Alternating
Shock wave	Present	Absent
Flashover	Present	Not prominent
Cardiac	Asystole	Fibrillation
Burns	Superficial, minor	Deep
Urinary failure	Rare myoglobinuria and hemoglobinuria	Myoglobinuric renal failure (common)
Fasciotomy and amputation	Rarely, if ever, necessary	Common, early, and extensive

Modified from Cooper, M. A., in *Management of Wilderness and Environmental Emergencies,* Auerbach, P. et al., Eds., Macmillan, New York, 1983.

Kleinot et al.[5] report similar findings in two cases, but in their first case with added ST elevation in I, aVL, and V_1 to V_4 and with depression in III, aVR, and aVF. T-wave inversion occurred anteriorly. The damage was thought to be anterior and epicardial. In the second case, the damage was inferior. In both cases, no Q-waves were seen, and complete regression of all changes occurred.

Chia,[17] on the other hand, reported ECG abnormalities of the ischemic type with diffuse T-wave inversion. Burda[6] reports similarly, as does Zeana[8] and Subramanian et al.[9] (see Figure 2). Coupled with the T-wave changes, ST segment "coving" has often been reported.

Jackson[15] presents two cases simulating myocardial necrosis and infarction, but with normal thallium uptake. Complete regression also occurred.

ECG abnormalities may not be evident on presentation and may develop subsequently[7,8] over periods varying to several days. Indeed, Zeana[8] reports the appearance of abnormalities on day 2, their disappearance, and subsequent reappearance on day 7 (Figures 2 and 3).

P-wave abnormalities have been reported,[6] including flattening and subsequent notching to biphasicity, but not widening.

Lengthening of the Q-T interval has been noted, with shortening in later development.[6] Palmer[10] reports developing Q-T lengthening, with deep inferior T-wave changes developing over 2 to 4 d and slowly regressing.

Kleiner and Wilkin[11] present a case of ischemic pattern injury, complicated in quick succession by acute pulmonary edema, but with normal cardiac size. Catheterization at 6 weeks showed diffuse LV hypokinesis with an ejection fraction of 47%. Filling pressures and selective arteriograms were normal. At $2^1/_2$ months, exercise tolerance was normal as measured by the treadmill test.

Cardiac enzyme levels generally show a small rise,[15,16] but caution is necessary[15] in interpreting CK levels in the presence of skeletal muscle trauma. Harwood et al.[16] draw attention to instances of brain-CK enzyme rise and document the case of a lightning-injured boy demonstrating this phenomenon. Brain injury is often present in lightning strike. McCarthy and Parker[56] reported a case with massive CK rise, and Ekoe et al.[55] reported a case where severe myocardial necrosis was seen at post-mortem.

Transient hypertension and tachycardia have been reported,[11,14] possibly due to a hyperadrenergic state.[17] These features are not uncommon, however, in any patient with a cerebral injury. Cardiac failure has also been reported.[17]

With regard to the vascular system, an unusual transient paralysis of limbs in the current path

TABLE 3
Finding Frequencies from Post-Mortem Examinations (10 cases)
Queensland, Australia, 1935–1988

Years	1941, 1945, 1961, 1964, 1965, 1967(2), 1968, 1975, 1985
Months	January (4), February (1), October (2), Novermber (3)
Sex	Male (8), female (2)
Situation	Sport/recreation (5), home (1), vagrant (1), work (2), indoor (1)
Bystanders	In six cases, bystanders (including a pet cockatoo in a struck tree) were affected; all recovered
Abrasions/burns	10/10, mostly in line of current arc (specifically, 2 said to be arborescent; 1 related to coins in pocket)
Singed hair	7/10, mostly cranial and pubic
Clothing damage	3/10, including one shattered wooden leg
Heart	No macroscopic damage in any case; in one case, LV systole, with RV diastole
Respiratory	6/10, lungs congested with/without frank edema
GI	3/9, hepatic congestion 1/9, intestinal congestion 3/9, splenic congestion
Renal	1/9, renal/suprarenal congestion
Cranium	1/9, congested cerebrum 5/9, intracranial-extracerebral bleeding 3/9, scalp hemorrhage 2/9, basal ganglion/thalamic hemorrhage (1/9, intracerebral hemorrhage in addition) 1/9, fractured skull
Mechanism	5/10, splash 4/10, direct (including 1 on water) 1/10, not recorded

Note: m/n represent m occurrences of the finding in n cases where explicit mention of the involved system was made.

The cooperation of Dr. A. Ansford, director, and staff, Queensland Institute of Forensic Pathology, in providing access to material for this table is acknowledged.

may be seen. This paralysis is a flaccid paralysis, with the appendage being cold, pulseless, cyanotic, and anesthetic. This "keraunoparalysis" is further discussed in Chapter 6 by ten Duis, but is documented here since one theory of its genesis invokes vascular spasm. It is a transient phenomenon[18] which resolves completely within 24 h, but is easily confused with a compartment syndrome.

B. RESPIRATORY SYSTEM
The respiratory system is intimately associated with the cardiovascular system, so that both may be affected by lightning injury. In particular, the respiratory system may suffer an arrest at

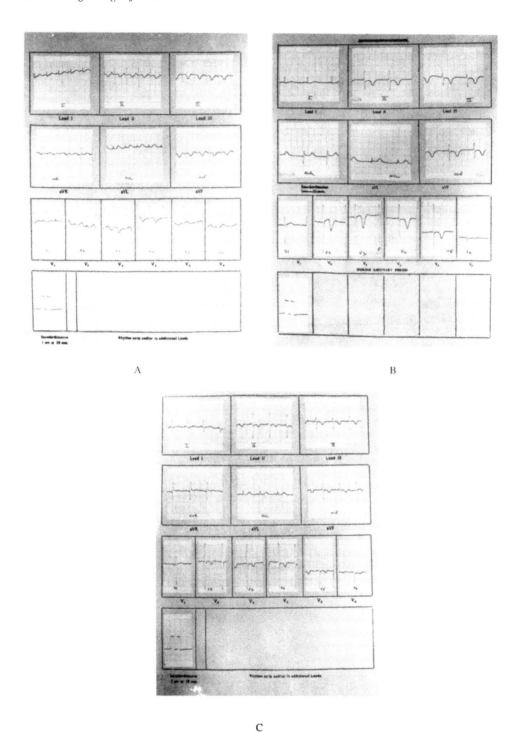

A   B

C

FIGURE 1. Electrocardiographic changes of infarction. T-wave inversion and ST segment elevation is seen, indicating possible cardiac muscle death. (From Sinha, A. K., *Angiology,* 36, 327, 1985. With permission.)

the same time as the cardiac arrest. The neurologic control center for the respiratory system, including the lungs and the muscles and nerves which control them, is located in the brainstem, which can be affected by the lightning stroke. Often, the respiratory arrest lasts longer than the cardiac arrest and may be responsible for the secondary cardiac arrest that is hypothesized to

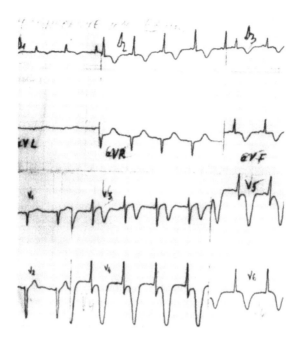

FIGURE 2. Electrocardiographic changes of ischemia 7 d post-injury. Diffuse T-wave inversion and ST segment depression is seen, indicating possible cardiac muscle embarrassment for oxygen. (From Zeana, C. D., *Int. J. Cardiol.*, 51, 207, 1984. With permission.)

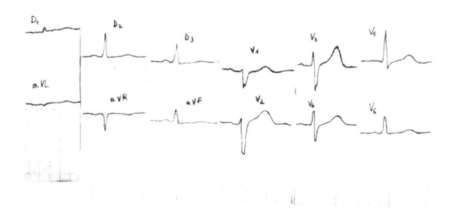

FIGURE 3. Electrocardiographic changes of ischemia, 7 months post-injury. Diffuse T-wave inversion and ST segment depression is seen, indicating possible cardiac muscle embarrassment for oxygen. (From Zeana, C. D., *Int. J. Cardiol.*, 51, 207, 1984. With permission.)

occur when the heart, which may have started beating again, does not receive adequate oxygenation to continue its function.

Other specifically pulmonary injuries reported are few, but include pulmonary edema, "bronchospasm", and contusion attributable to the "blast" associated with the lightning discharge.[21] Surgical emphysema has also been found.[21]

IV. NEUROLOGICAL SYSTEM
(Contributed by M. J. Eadie)

A. ACUTE NEUROLOGICAL DISTURBANCES

Perusal of the literature suggests that there are two main clinical patterns of acute neurological disorder associated with lightning strike. In the first, lightning strike causes abrupt loss of consciousness. The interruption of consciousness may be quite brief, or last for minutes, hours, or days. The victim lies immobile, without the twitchings or convulsions that are common in electrocution injuries, although incontinence of urine and/or ejaculation of semen may occur. Commonly, there is cessation of heart action and breathing, so that the victim appears clinically dead. This cardiorespiratory arrest may be the result of an electrically induced medullary disturbance and/or direct myocardial depolarization. However, if artificial respiration is instituted at this stage, there are reasonable prospects that spontaneous cardiac and respiratory activity will return,[1,2] followed by recovery of consciousness. The degree of neurological recovery possible after many minutes of apparent total cardiorespiratory arrest has led to speculation that lightning strike in humans may lead to something akin to a state of suspended animation.[2,20] Conceivably, massive cerebral depolarization decreases cerebral metabolic activity to an extent that permits unusually long survival of neurons in the face of anoxia. There may be a full period of disorientation and confusion during the return of full consciousness.

Amnesia for the event is common[25] and can include both retrograde and anterograde components. The person struck commonly reports only some sensation of a dull blow. The statement "The man who sees the lightning and hears the thunder is not the one who is struck" has been attributed to Pliny and Elder.[29] As indicated in the post-mortem review of Table 3, intracranial hemorrhage is perhaps more common than reported, with the basal ganglia and cerebellum often being affected (see Table 3 and Reference 28).

Immediately after the lightning strike, there may be a variety of temporary and sometimes enduring pupillary abnormalities. These include dilated, nonreacting pupils (which in the presence of cardiorespiratory arrest may be mistakenly interpreted as indicating irretrievable brain death[33]), Horner's syndrome, anisocoria, and pupillary myotonia. There may also be temporary sensory symptoms, e.g., painful paresthesiae, particularly involving the limbs.[26] The majority of victims of lightning injury who regain consciousness are left with no long-term neurological sequelae, but temporary or permanent neurological disorders may occur, e.g., decerebrate rigidity,[66] aphasia,[30] and headache. All the latter may exist in the absence of abnormal neurological signs.[30,35,67] Delayed onset neurological sequelae (to be discussed below) may develop occasionally. Autonomic neuropathy, i.e., disturbances in unconscious automatic body functions due to damage to the nerves controlling them, may be found.[30,63]

The second major pattern of acute neurological disturbance resulting from lightning strike is the so-called "keraunoparesis", first described by Charcot (1889). This pattern of disturbance usually appears to be associated with the stride potential situation. Initially, there is often a period of loss of consciousness, although usually brief and without associated cardiorespiratory arrest. Once consciousness returns, the victim proves to have an areflexic flaccid paresis of the lower limbs, in which the arterial pulses are impalpable. Over the next few hours, in general contemporaneous with the return of the arterial pulses in the legs, power returns to the lower limbs so that, usually within a day or two, there is no detectable neurological residue. Occasionally, the paraparesis may persist[66] or there may be continuing neuritic and paresthetic symptoms.[30]

Other less common patterns of immediate neurological dysfunction have been described in relation to lightning injury. A lightning strike may be conducted to the side of the head via the telephone system if the victim is holding a telephone to his or her ear when the current strikes the system (see Reference 68 and Appendix 1). In this situation, as well as the burn injury

centered on the ear to which the phone is held and the frequent rupture of the ipsilateral tympanic membrane, there may sometimes be a delayed onset facial nerve palsy, also on the same side.[52] During a storm, a lightning strike may be transmitted via an opened umbrella to the victim's hand. One such instance was followed by a median nerve palsy on that side.[69] The report did not contain sufficient detail to determine whether the injury was a direct electrical effect or was due to nerve compression, possibly from associated ischemic muscle swelling in the forearm, or had some other explanation. Peters[70] described reversible muscle wasting and weakness in one arm of the victim of a lightning strike.

B. DELAYED ONSET NEUROLOGICAL DISTURBANCE

As mentioned above, in the great majority of instances, if the victim survives, the severe neurological disturbance of the acute phase of lightning injury is followed by full or nearly full recovery. In a minority of instances of lightning strike, delayed onset neurological disturbances may occur after earlier apparent recovery. These disturbances have included epileptic seizures,[26,30] inappropriate ADH secretion,[36] progressive hemiparesis due to an extradural hematoma[3] which was itself due to a head injury when the victim was thrown to the ground, and myelopathy beginning 36 h after the strike and producing an incompletely reversible pyramidal tract deficit in the lower limbs.[31] Langworthy[71] described a patient who developed a right hemiparesis of 24-h duration after a lightning strike. After 3 weeks, a tremor developed in this subject's right arm, with loss of associated movement in the arm. Damage to the left basal ganglia was postulated.[72] Other instances of the Parkinsonian-type syndrome associated with lightning injury are known.[73] Although several papers have mentioned the development of spinal atrophic paresis as a delayed sequel of lightning injury and Panse,[73] in his review, described several reports of this event, the original literature more often associates this phenomenon with electrocution than with lightning strike. Myers et al.[66] did record a comparatively recent instance following lightning strike, but the details were scanty. Leys[74] described an earlier instance in which a lightning strike was followed within days by the progressive development of atrophic paresis of the upper limbs, associated with muscle fasciculation. The subsequent evolution of the disorder resembled that of the progressive muscular atrophy variety of motor neuron disease.

V. PSYCHIATRIC SYMPTOMATOLOGY

Many changes in the psychiatric functioning of the patient have been reported. Critchley[29] gave the first "modern" description of these effects and noted that consciousness is nearly always lost, but the loss rarely lasts for more than 2 h. While Critchley disagrees, most authorities accept that retrograde amnesia is common.

Anterograde amnesia is also commonly seen for the first few days, and the victim closely resembles a patient who has had electroconvulsive shock therapy for severe depression.

In initial recovery, Critchley[29] noted states of noisy excitement with restlessness and anxiety, and even convulsions.[30] Kotogal et al.[26] report similarly. Disturbed sleep was common in Critchley's cases, and a strange flat disinterest was seen in some, while a state of considerable agitation was seen in others. Indeed, it was reported that this state took up to a week to subside, with crying and anxiety, coupled with a state of extreme self-interest and nonconcern about others possibly injured. A state of fugue, and also of "suspended animation", has also been reported.

The physical signs of various paralyses, blindness, deafness, etc. seen soon after the strike are reported to be examples of degrees of hysteria, and subsequent reemergence at times of stress has also been said to be hysterical. On the other hand, some have said that these paralyses are specifically organic, and, indeed, Charcot coined the name "keraunoparalysis", now applied to the specific entity described elsewhere in this volume. Nonetheless, functionally based deficits are often seen.

In the long term, Critchley[29] identifies confusional states and depressive psychoses. He also reports other psychoses, including atypical manic depression[35] and a paranoid psychosis. Also reported are hypochondriasis, agoraphobia, and long-term depression.[35] On the other hand, beneficial effects of a stroke have been reported, and reports of psychotic illness and hysterical illness both improving after lightning shock have been given.[30] Whether or not post-strike disorders can be ascribed to lightning, or to exacerbation of preexisting pathology, is debated.

Shaw and York-Moore[35] foreshadow a modern resurgence of interest in "post-traumatic neurosis" and ascribe many of the hysterical and neurotic symptoms to this causation. Bach (in Reference 25) described a post-traumatic syndrome, although with dilated ventricles demonstrated on investigation. Shaw and York-Moore[35] place psychiatric symptomatology after the Ascot incident in context in the following figures, derived from the follow-up of Ascot and Aldershot victims:

Symptom	Effects (%)	
	Early	Late
Headache	34	11
Paralysis (all causes)	25	4
Anxiety/hysteria	19	11
Fatigue	12	0
Deafness (all causes)	9	4
Dysphasia (all causes)	6	0
Depression	3	7

Kotogal, et al.[26] documented one case as follows:

> ... the patient developed frequent episodes of denial of the accident, marked agitation, and crying. He became emotionally labile and very often expressed a fear of dying. This alternated with periods of depression. These disturbances of mood and behavior gradually resolved over the ensuing months with supportive psychotherapy.

This seems a useful report, and in the present authors' view, early psychiatric intervention with a focus on preventive interviewing may alleviate later problems.

Little has been written on cognitive function, but Frayne et al.[23] note a patient demonstrating a marked discrepancy between verbal and nonverbal memory, with difficulty learning new, complex material. In addition, personality change incorporating aggression and verbal abuse occurred with swinging mood. A second patient showed reduced concentration, with some loss in problem-solving ability and slowed coordination. Both patients' problems resolved gradually.

VI. OCULAR SYMPTOMATOLOGY

The eyes are particularly vulnerable to injury from electric current, and, indeed, it has been pointed out[19,62] that this may be more important than previously thought. The ocular media are relatively well conducting, and via the lacrimal apparatus may provide a portal of entry to the pharynx and possibly to the cervical cord.[62] Pfahl (quoted in Reference 42) states that 55% of lightning victims show eye involvement.

Early signs of eye damage include corneal flash burns, somewhat akin to welder's flash, and punctate keratitis. Photophobia and eye pain associated with inflammation and edema of all external media are not uncommon.[37] Burns, thermal and lightning current induced, are, of course, common.[36-38] Vitreous hemorrhage, iridocylitis, retinal tear, macular puncture, and

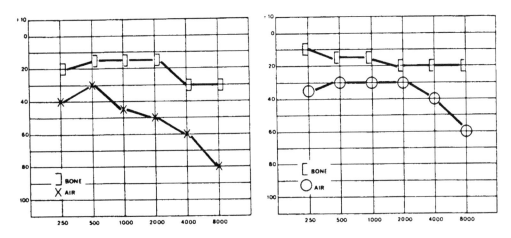

FIGURE 4. Audiograms from two patients with lightning-induced conductive deafness. (From Kristensen, S. and Tveteras, K., *J. Laryngol. Otol.*, 99, 711, 1985. With permission.)

retinal detachment have all been reported.[37-39,41-44] Visual field defect, mostly scotomatous, has also been noted,[39] and a postulated sympathetic autoimmune uveitis has been documented.[40]

One particularly important aspect of the lightning-injured eye is the possibility of various ocular pareses which can occur, locally mediated. These may be autonomic[37] or skeletal,[41] and need to be borne in mind specifically when interpreting ocular signs of brain stem function. It has been strongly noted that such signs are acutely unreliable.

Longer-term complications are important with ocular injuries, and the most common is the induction of cataract formation (see review in Reference 36). Fraunfelder discusses these injuries in considerable detail elsewhere in this volume.

Long-term retinitis and optic neuritis (with or without papilloedema), macular degeneration, optic atrophy, and neuroplegia are also important. Persistent loss of color vision of a deuteranope type has also been reported.[42]

VII. COCHLEOVESTIBULAR SYMPTOMS

The otological apparatus is also vulnerable to insult, and in addition to electrical and thermal damage, may sustain acoustic damage akin to barotrauma. Ruptured tympanic membrane, with deafness and otorrhea, is therefore common.[45] Kristensen states that the level of insult can reach 155 dB SPL. Bergstrom discusses these problems in more detail in Chapter 6. Ossicular damage by blast trauma is also possible, resulting in conductive deafness, particularly at high frequency. Figure 4 shows audiograms of two patients with conductive deafness due to lightning trauma.

Middle ear injury has been reviewed by Bellucci,[46] and can be caused directly, with injury transmitted through the external canal or as a secondary consequence of skull trauma, including fracture. These injuries are common and may be made manifest[50-52] by symptoms and signs related to tympanic membrane, ossicular chain, facial nerve, and oval and round windows.

Inner ear damage is manifest through neural hearing signs or labrynthine signs, although less common than conductive damage. Ataxia, deafness, and nystagmus are cardinal findings, with accompanying nausea, tinnitus, and pain.[46,48,49,51] An audiogram and the cruder tuning fork tests help to differentiate the localization.[47]

Burns in all these areas are commonly seen, as are hemorrhage and inflammation. Frank otitis media, possibly as a consequence of perforation, has also been seen,[50] but is rare. Organization of a hematoma with calcification, producing a space-occupying lesion, has been noted.[53]

Stated in summary form like this, the list of otological symptoms is small, and yet these injuries account for significant morbidity. This problem is particularly marked with telephone-mediated strike.

VIII. RENAL, GASTROINTESTINAL, HEMATOLOGIC, AND ENDOCRINE SYMPTOMS

Many findings with regard to these systems have been reported, but often in isolated reports.

Myoglobinuria, so common after massive muscle trauma via "technical" electricity, is only reported in passing with regard to lightning injury. When it does occur, it seems to cause little problem compared with its catastrophic consequences with other injuries. Yost and Holmes[54] report the phenomenon in the only paper dedicated to the topic. Macroscopic hematuria with casts, clumps, and myoglobin was found. These cleared by day 3 to 5. Creatine phosphokinase (CPK), lactate dehydrogenase (LDH), and serum glutamic oxaloacetic transaminase (SGOT) were all grossly elevated, reflecting severe damage.

Hematological findings are rare. Ekoe et al.[55] report DIC in a patient with cardiogenic shock after being resuscitated from cardiorespiratory arrest and exhibiting 20% "second-degree" burns. McCarthy and Parker[56] report the transient appearance of positive direct and indirect antiglobin tests. This report is the only one in the area, and the effect must be regarded as rare. CPK was again massively elevated.

Eng and Sinnadurai[57] report a bizarre case of a man in good health struck by lightning. After the strike, he was unable to work due to generalized weakness. Subsequently, he became pale and edematous, and was found to be anemic. Autoimmune hemolysis was demonstrated. Marrow hyperactivity resembling that in the di Guglielmo syndrome was also seen. Over 1 month, the patient deteriorated, and toward the time of his death, changes of acute monocytic leukemia were seen. This latter progression is known in other circumstances, and it is possible that the lightning strike might have initiated the initial autoimmune process, with the natural course of progression ensuing. This remains speculative, however.

Reference has already been made to the hyperadrenergic state said to exist after lightning strike, giving rise to hypertension and tachycardia.

Alcock and Fletcher-Jones[58] and Milward[59] describe cases of abdominal injury. Gangrenous areas of bowel were described, with ileus in one case and prolonged gastric dilatation in another. Ehsan et al.[60] describe a delayed case of well-demarcated gangrene similar to that seen as a result of progressive vascular occlusion. There was no evidence, however, of vasculitis on histology.

IX. MUSCULOSKELETAL SYSTEM

The syndrome of keraunoparalysis is described by ten Duis (see Chapter 6). In addition, traumatic musculoskeletal injury is seen in all its forms, with evidence variously of contusions, lacerations, and fractures of bones, including skull and spine. Contusion of lung, heart, and gut, possibly due to pressure effects, has been described.

X. BURNS

Of great interest are the burns seen in lightning injury. Their appearance (shown in Figures 5 to 10) allows classification into six main groups, although Hocking and Andrews[61] have suggested that three (arborescent, linear, and erythema) are all manifestations of the same phenomenon. ten Duis (see Chapter 6) deals with this in more detail. The classification is

1. Flash burns
2. Feathering — "arborescent" burns
3. Erythema and blistering — "flower-like" burns
4. Linear streaking
5. Punctate full-thickness skin loss
6. Contact burn from metal

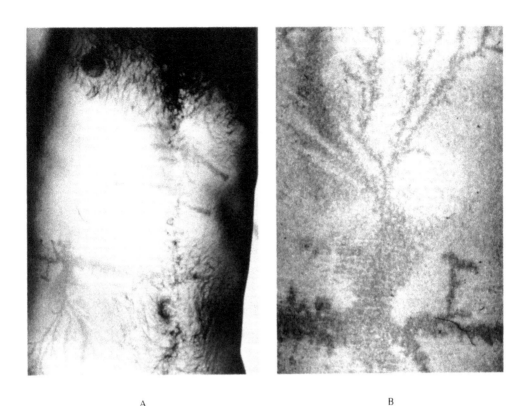

A   B

FIGURE 5. Arborescent burns. (Courtesy of Dr. B. Hocking.)

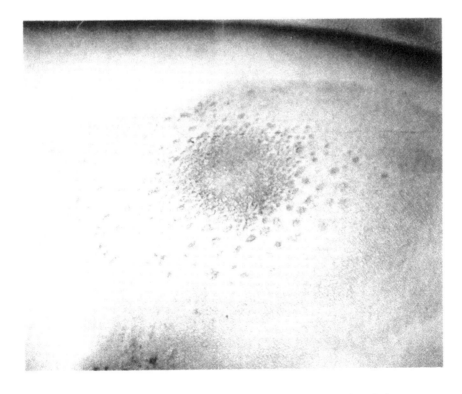

FIGURE 6. Erythematous (flower-like) burns. (Courtesy of Dr. H. J. ten Duis.)

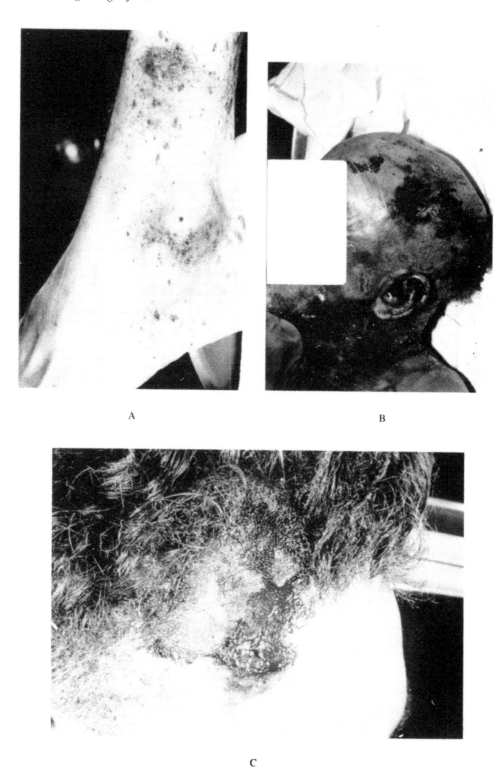

A

B

C

FIGURE 7. Punctate (A) and full-thickness burns (B, C) at entry/exit sites. (7B courtesy of Dr. S. Kristensen.)

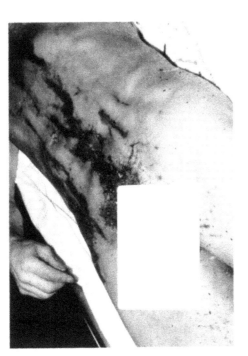

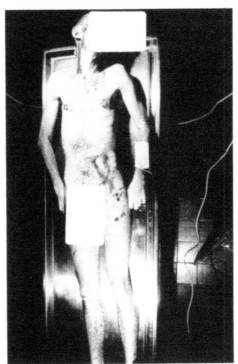

A   B

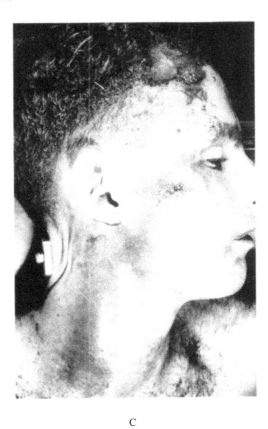

C

FIGURE 8. Linear burns. (8A courtesy of Dr. S. Kristensen.)

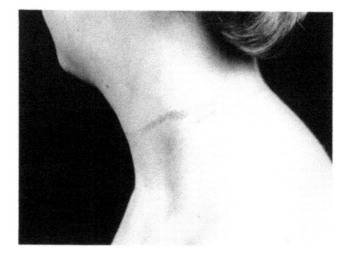

A

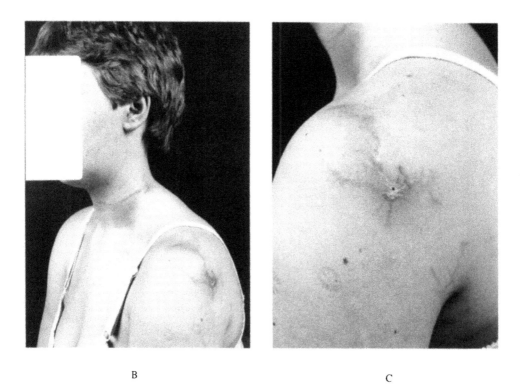

B   C

FIGURE 9. (A) Contact burns from metal apparel; (B, C) also showing entry burn and detail with arborescent track. (Courtesy of Dr. S. Kristensen.)

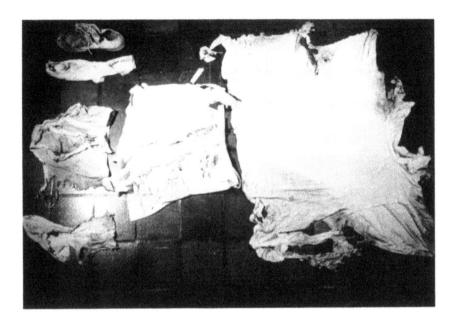

FIGURE 10. Clothing damage caused by lightning strike. Man struck while playing cricket, Brisbane, 1961.

The feathering type of burn appears as a linear superficial skin marking which is transient and disappears within a few days. Its pattern is arborescent and branching, and it does not blanche on pressure. It has been called a "keraunic marking". These markings are analogous to the Lichtenberg figure well known to electrical engineers. Bartholome (1975) describes these as "bizarre, superficial erythema". It is said that these are pathognomonic of lightning injury and may be of great diagnostic importance in a comatose patient.

Flash burns may be thought of as analogous to those received by welders when they report welder's flash. Flash burns are generally quite superficial and usually exhibit only erythema and sometimes mild blistering. They often spare the crease lines, but may include the cornea, on occasion. Skin loss is uncommon.

Punctate full-thickness skin burns may occur, but are uncommon. They usually appear as small areas that are similar to cigarette burns in size and appearance and may either be isolated or in a group, sometimes in concentric rings of decreasing-size spots. They are particularly characteristic of current entry and exit burns.

Linear burns occur as strips of burnt skin ranging from a few millimeters to 5 cm. They are usually partial thickness and do not result in major skin loss. They sometimes occur in groups and other times occur along the sweat lines of a patient, involving the mid-axillary line or the center of the chest in long lines down the torso, sometimes splitting to go down each leg.

Contact burns are from metal that is worn close to the skin, such as zippers, necklaces, and pocket coins, that become heated from the flow of lightning current over the body. They can be full-thickness burns and may need grafting, depending on their size.

While deep burns, similar to those caused by exposure to high-voltage, man-made, electrical systems have been occasionally reported, they are rare.

XI. DIFFERENTIAL DIAGNOSIS AND FORENSIC SIGNIFICANCE

Cooper[65] has examined these topics in detail. This chapter concludes with an excerpt from that work.

The diagnosis of lightning injury is sometimes difficult to make. Often there is a history of a thunderstorm, witnesses who can report having seen the strike, and typical physical findings in the victim.

However, lightning can strike on an apparently sunny day and thunder may not be appreciated.

If the victim is struck while working alone in a field, the diagnosis may be initially confused with several other processes, including ruptured cerebral aneurysm or another cerebral vascular accident, seizure disorder, spinal cord injury, closed head injury, Stokes-Adams attack or another arrhythmia, hypertensive crisis with intracerebral hemorrhage, myocardial infarction, or toxin ingestion (particularly of heavy metals).

In the past, persons have been thought to be the victims of an assault, because of the disarray of their belongings and clothing damage. The history and a careful physical examination at the earliest opportunity can be very helpful in differentiating the true cause. This is of obvious forensic importance.

Any person found in the open with linear burns and his clothes exploded off should be treated as a victim of lightning strike. Feathering burns are pathognomonic of lightning strike and occur in no other type of injury. Unfortunately, they are not always present in lightning victims. Another complex that is diagnostic of lightning strike includes linear or punctate burns, tympanic membrane rupture, confusion, and being found in the open whether or not there is a history of a thunderstorm.

XII. DECLARATION OF DEATH

Somewhere between 20 and 30% of lightning victims die because of their injuries. The vast majority of these die at the time of the strike and are nonresuscitatable. The few who die after resuscitation and prolonged care must have appropriate criteria employed for pronouncement of death.

For the most part, standard criteria for brain death, such as lack of spontaneous movement, spontaneous respirations, and deep tendon reflexes, can be used in determining brain death. Other significant signs include failure to maintain body temperature, and EEG silence. Pupillary functions and other cranial nerve signs cannot be used reliably to determine death, since they may be directly affected by the lightning stroke and not functioning properly.

REFERENCES

1. **Ravitch, M. M., Lane, R., Safar, P., Steichen, F., and Knowles, P.,** Lightning stroke, *N. Engl. J. Med.,* 264, 36, 1961.
2. **Taussig, H.,** 'Death' from lightning and the possibility of living again, *Ann. Int. Med.,* 68, 1345, 1968.
3. **Morgan, Z. V., Headley, R. N., Alexander, E. A., and Sawyer, C. G.,** Atrial fibrillation and epidural haematoma associated with lightning stroke, *N. Engl. J. Med.,* 259, 956, 1958.
4. **Sinha, A. K.,** Lightning induced myocardial injury — a case report with management, *Angiology,* 36, 327, 1985.
5. **Kleinot, S., Klachko, D. M., and Keeley, K. J.,** The cardiac effects of lightning injury, *S. Afr. Med. J.,* 40, 1141, 1966.
6. **Burda, C. A.,** Electrocardiographic changes in lightning stroke, *Am. Heart. J.,* 72, 521, 1966.
7. **Read, J. M.,** Man struck by lightning reveals marked ECG changes hours later, *Med. Trib.,* p. 3, March 28, 1966.
8. **Zeana, C. D.,** Acute transient myocardial ischaemia after lightning injury, *Int. J. Cardiol.,* 5, 207, 1984.
9. **Subramanian, N.,** Cardiac injury due to lightning — report of a survivor, *Indian Heart J.,* 37(1), 72, 1985.

10. **Palmer, A. B. D.,** Lightning injury causing prolongation of the Q-T internal, *Postgrad. Med. J.,* 63, 891, 1987.
11. **Kleiner, J. P. and Wilkin, J. H.,** Cardiac effects of lightning stroke, *JAMA,* 240, 2757, 1978.
12. **Yost, J. W. and Holmes, F. F.,** Myoglobinuria following lightning stroke", *JAMA.* 228, 1147, 1974.
13. **Hansen, G. C. and McIlwraith, G. R.,** Lightning injury: two case histories and a review of management, *Br. Med. J.,* 4, 271, 1973.
14. **Kravitz, H., Wasserman, M. J., Valaitis, J., et al.,** Lightning injury, *Am. J. Dis. Child.,* 131, 413, 1977.
15. **Jackson, S. H. D.,** Lightning and the heart, *Br. Heart. J.,* 43, 454, 1980.
16. **Harwood, S. J., Catrou, R. G., and Cole, G. W.,** Creatine phosphokinase isoenzyme fractions in the serum of a patient struck by lightning, *Arch. Int. Med.,* 138, 645, 1978.
17. **Chia, B. L.,** Electrocardiographic abnormalities and congestive cardiac failure due to lightning stroke, *Cardiology,* 68, 49, 1981.
18. **Currens, J. H.,** Arterial spasm and transient paralysis from lightning striking an aeroplane, *Aerosp. Med.,* formerly *Aviat. Med.,* 16, 275, 1945.
19. **Andrews, C. J., and Darveniza, M.,** Lightning injury — a review of clinical aspects, pathophysiology and treatment, *Adv. Trauma,* 4, 241, 1989.
20. **Apfelberg, D. B., Masters, F. W., and Robinson, D. W.,** Pathophysiology of treatment of lightning injuries, *J. Trauma,* 14(6), 453, 1974.
21. **Moulson, A. M.,** Blast injury of the lungs due to lightning, *Br. Med. J.,* 289, 1270, 1984.
22. **Draper, P. A.,** Neuropsychiatric effects of electric trauma, *Col. Med.,* September, 650, 1937.
23. **Frayne, J. and Gilligan, B. S.,** Neurological sequelae of lightning stroke, *Clin. Exp. Neurol.,* 24, 195, 1988.
24. **Suri, M. L. and Vijayan, G. P.,** Neurological sequelae of lightning, *J. Assoc. Phys. Ind.,* 26, 209, 1978.
25. **Gathier, J. C.,** Neurological changes in a soldier hit by lightning, *Psychiatr. Neurol. Neurochir.,* 63, 125, 1960.
26. **Kotogal, S., Rawlings, C. A., Chen, S., Burris, G., and Nouri, S.,** Neurologic, psychiatric and cardiovascular complications in children struck by lightning, *Paediatrics,* 70(2), 190, 1982.
27. **Paterson, J. H. and Turner, J. W.,** Lightning and the central nervous system, *J. R. Army Med. Corps,* 82, 73, 1944.
28. **Wakasugi, C. and Masui, M.,** Secondary brain hemorrhages associated with lightning stroke: report of a case, *Jpn. J. Legal Med.,* 40(1), 42, 1986.
29. **Critchley, M.,** The effects of lightning with especial reference to the nervous system, *Bristol Med. Chir. J.,* 49, 285, 1932.
30. **Critchley, M.,** Neurological effects of lightning and of electricity, *Lancet,* 1, 68, 1934.
31. **Sharma, M. et al.,** Paraplegia as a result of lightning injury, *Br. Med. J.,* 25 Nov. 1978, p. 1464.
32. **Stanley, L. D. and Suss, R. A.,** Intracerebral haematoma secondary to lightning stroke: case report and review of literature, *Neurosurgery,* 16, 686, 1985.
33. **Abt, J. L.,** The pupillary responses after being struck by lightning, *JAMA,* 254, 3312, 1985.
34. **Mann, H., Kozic, Z., and Boulos, M.,** CT of lightning injury, *Am. J. Neuroradiol.,* 4, 976, 1983.
35. **Shaw, D. and York-Moore, M.,** Neuropsychiatric sequelae of lightning stroke, *Br. Med. J.,* 2, 1152, 1957.
36. **Shapiro, M. B.,** Lightning cataracts, *Wis. Med. J.,* 83, 23, 1984.
37. **Lea, J. A.,** Paresis of accommodation following injury by lightning, *Br. J. Ophthalmol.,* 4, 417, 1920.
38. **Du Toit, J. S.,** Lightning injury, *Can. Med. Assoc., J.,* 128, 893, 1983.
39. **Moore, M. C.,** Ocular injury from lightning current and lightning flash, *Trans. Ophthalmol. Soc. Aust.,* 16, 87, 1956.
40. **Raymond, L. F.,** Specific treatment of uveitis, lightning induced: an autoimmune disease, *Ann. Allerg.,* 27, 242, 1967.
41. **Sheppard, L. B.,** Report of an eye injured by lightning, *Am. J. Ophthalmol.,* 28, 195, 1945.
42. **Castren, J. A. and Kytila, J.,** Eye symptoms caused by lightning, *Acta Ophthalmol.,* 41, 139, 1963.
43. **Noel, L. P., Clarke, W. N., and Addison, D.,** Ocular complications of lightning, *J. Paediatr. Opthalmol.,* 17, 245, 1980.
44. **Campo, R. V.,** Lightning induced macular hole, *Am. J. Ophthalmol.,* 97, 792, 1984.
45. **Kristensen, S. and Tveteras, K.,** Lightning induced acoustic rupture of the tympanic membrane, *J. Laryngol. Otol.,* 99, 711, 1985.
46. **Bellucci, R. J.,** Traumatic injuries of the middle ear, *Otolaryngol. Clin. N. Am.,* 16, 633, 1983.
47. **Weiss, K. S.,** Otological lightning bolts, *Am. J. Otol.,* 1, 334, 1980.
48. **Spirov, A.,** Damage of the ear by thunderbolt, *Vojnosanit. Pregl.,* 25(12), 648, 1968.
49. **Gusakov, A. D. and Zaiko, N. G.,** Lesion of the human middle ear caused by lightning, *Zh. Ushn. Nos. Gorl. Bolez.,* 5, 67, 1979.
50. **West, G.,** Lightning as a cause of hearing loss, *Md. State. Med. J.,* 4, 35, 1955.
51. **Wright, J. W. et al.,** Acoustic and vestibular defects in lightning survivors, *Laryngoscope,* 84, 1378, 1974.
52. **Richards, A.,** Traumatic facial palsy, *Proc. R. Soc. Med.,* 66, 28, 1973.

53. **Poulsen, P. and Knudstrup, P.,** Lightning caused inner ear damage and intracranial haematoma, *J. Laryngol. Otol.,* 100, 1067, 1986.

54. **Yost, J. W. and Holmes, F. F.,** Myoglobinuria following lightning stroke, *JAMA,* 228, 1147, 1974.

55. **Ekoe, J. M., Cunningham, M., Jaques, O., et al.,** Disseminated intravascular coagulation and acute myocardial necrosis caused by lightning, *Int. Care Med.,* 11, 160, 1985.

56. **McCarthy, L. J. and Parker, C.,** Positive antiglobulin tests in a boy struck by lightning, *N. Engl. J. Med.,* 305, 283, 1987.

57. **Eng, L. and Sinnadurai, C.,** Syndrome of Erythemia di Guglielmo after lightning injury with autoimmune antibodies and terminating in acute monocytic leukaemia, *Blood,* 25, 845, 1965.

58. **Alcock, R. and Fletcher-Jones, H. C.,** Abdominal injury from lightning, *Lancet,* 1, 823, 1949.

59. **Milward, J. M.,** Prolonged gastric dilatation as a complication of lightning injury, *Burns,* 1, 175, 1975.

60. **Ehsan, M., Waxman, J., and Finley, J. M.,** Delayed gangrene after lightning strike, *A.F.P.,.* 24, 117, 1981.

61. **Hocking, B. and Andrews, C. J.,** Fractals and lightning injury, *Med. J. Aust.,* 150(7), 409, 1989.

62. **Andrews, C. and Darveniza, M.,** Effect of lightning strike on mammalian tissue, in Proc 3rd Int. Conf. Lightning and Static Electricity, ERA Technology, Surrey, U.K., 1989.

63. **Weeramanthri, T.,** personal communication.

64. **Cooper, M. A.,** Lightning injuries: prognostic signs for death, *Ann. Emerg. Med.,* 9, 134, 1980.

65. **Cooper, M. A.,** Lightning injuries, in *Management of Wilderness and Environmental Emergencies,* Auerbach, P. et al., Eds., MacMillan, New York, 1983.

66. **Myers, G. J., Colgan, M. J., and Van Dyck, D. H.,** Lightning strike disaster among children, *JAMA,* 238, 1045, 1977.

67. **Strasser, E. J. et al.,** Lightning injuries, *J. Trauma,* 17, 318, 1978.

68. **Johnstone, B. R., Harding, D. L., and Hocking, B.,** Telephone related lightning injury, *Med. J. Austr.,* 144, 706, 1986.

69. **Amy, B. W. et. al.,** Lightning injury with survival in five cases, *JAMA,* 253, 243, 1985.

70. **Peters, W. J.,** Lightning injury, *J. Can. Med. Assoc.,* 128, 148, 1983.

71. **Langworthy, O. R.,** Abnormalities produced in the central nervous system by electrical injuries, *J. Exp. Med.,* 51, 943, 1930.

72. **Farrell, D. F. and Starr, A.,** Delayed neurological sequelae of electrical injuries, *Neurology,* 18, 601, 1968.

73. **Panse, F.,** Electrical trauma, in *Handbook of Clinical Neurology,* Vinken, P. J. et. al., Eds., North Holland, Amsterdam, 23, 683, 1975.

74. **Leys, D.,** Spinal atrophic paralysis, *Edinburgh Med. J.,* 49, 657, 1942.

75. **Smith, J.,** Lightning injuries, *J. Emerg. Nurs.,* 9, 248, 1983.

76. **Arden, G., Harrison, S., Lister, J., and Maudsley, R.,** Lightning accident at Ascot, *Br. Med. J.,* June 23, 1450, 1956.

Chapter 6

PATHOPHYSIOLOGY OF LIGHTNING INJURY

My own idea is that, although death from lightning stroke is nearly allied to and closely resembles death by electricity, yet there is, on the one hand, something added, and on the other something absent. Of course, this is purely my opinion, and must be taken for what it is worth.

Oscar Dunscombe-Honiball
British Medical Journal, May 12, 1900

TABLE OF CONTENTS

I. INTRODUCTION

C. J. Andrews

In this chapter, the lesions thought to underlie the symptoms and signs of lightning injury are outlined. It is on the basis of these perceived lesions that rational treatment is given, and an enumeration of accepted modalities logically follows in Chapter 7.

Central to a discussion of pathophysiology are the mechanisms by which the lightning stroke affects the body. This is now examined.

In all lightning injury, one of several physical mechanisms operates, and conceivably combinations of these. Direct strike obviously portends the greatest damage, with stride potential due to earth potential rise (EPR) being the least harmful. Touch potential and "side-flash" impingement may be thought of as variants of direct strike, but of lesser magnitude. In considering injuries due to lightning strike, a model of the injuring agent and its impingement on the body is necessary. Accordingly, this section examines a model of the strike circumstance in an attempt to quantitate the insult to the victim.

The literature contains very little contemporary development of such a model. Blake-Pritchard[1] has already been referred to, and the remaining work on this facet of the subject has come from Japanese researchers, notably Ishikawa, Nagai, and Kitigawa. Their work has been aimed more at determining lethal levels of flash current and the relationship between the development of flashover and the lethality of a given flash.

Ishikawa et al.[2] examined the lethal current level of a flash to live unanesthetized rabbits using a multipulse technique. Their findings were that a threshold of approximately 62.6 J/kg existed, beyond which death would occur. Further, their finding was that provided one stroke in a multistroke flash exceeded this level, death would ensue. Specifically, there was no "memory" engendered for succeeding strokes, and no cumulative effect of multiple strokes was seen. The strokes were approximately 40 ms apart, three in number, and were applied directly to the animal's head via a needle. Energy input alone was examined, and no account was taken of synchrony with the cardiac cycle — especially the probability of transgressing the "vulnerable window" of late repolarization. Nagai et al.[3] confirmed the order of this energy level.

Ishikawa et al.[4] drew attention to the fact that if artificial ventilation was instituted after "death" from a lightning strike, survival was increased from 25 to 48%.

Ohashi et al.[5] also draw attention to the protective effect of the development of external flashover in a strike. Of 50 victims, 9 had evidence of flashover, and 41 showed no such evidence. Of the former, 5 survived, and the latter, only 6 survived. The division into groups was somewhat subjective, but nonetheless these results are striking. In an experimental determination, they noted two separate groups of animals subjected to artificial shocks. In those developing "early" flashover (sooner than 20 μs from contact), the survival was markedly better than in those developing later flashover. This was thought to be related to increased energy dissipation internally prior to flashover.

In a different approach, Flisowski[6] used an analytical technique to predict the mortality level from strikes given the probability distributions of stroke current, local parameters, and known fatal current levels for the human body. Although the latter are an extrapolation of Dalziel's well-known formula into regions of short impulses, the mortality level arrived at of 20 to 40% is of the order of that seen in practice. The body model used, however, was simply resistive, and took no account of reactive components and the different nature of the skin from the internal milieux.

A. EXPERIMENTAL PARALLELS

There are extreme experimental difficulties in verifying any of the above data on humans. It is unacceptable to subject human beings to shocks under laboratory conditions. This may be one reason why consideration of current pathways and magnitudes in humans has received so little attention.

An interesting parallel, however, exists in the work of Darveniza (Reference 7 and Chapter 3, q.v.), who examined the electrical properties of wood used in power reticulation structures. This biological material is markedly more homogeneous than the animal body, but nonetheless contains potential channels for internal breakdown that parallel the tissue planes and channel structures of the body.

Darveniza found that the breakdown path seen when a wooden structure was submitted to an impulse was either entirely internal or entirely external, never both. Which pathway was seen in an individual case was dependent on a number of factors, of which two were particularly important, viz., the moisture content of the wood (more moisture favoring the internal path) and the existence of an entry site (e.g., a bolt or the like) to the interior. In dry woods, moisture content less than 20%, the pathway was invariably external. In "wet" woods, moisture content greater than 50%, the pathway was invariably internal. In the intermediate range, other factors needed to be considered, such as length of wood sample, types of electrodes used, wet vs. dry surface conditions, and associated hardware.

Given this information, it is apparent that the human body has some features favoring truly internal breakdown. These include high moisture content, relatively short "length", and significant portals of entry. The latter include the special sense orifices of the cranium; more will be said of these later, representing significant findings of these orifices as more important portals of entry than previously thought, and hence also their vulnerability to injury. Nonetheless, the body possesses certain properties disposing to external flashover. These include the likelihood of being externally wet by rain, having less in the way of attached hardware such as bolts and screws, and being less homogeneous.

Darveniza notes that evidence of internal flashover in wood is often easily seen, as the internal pathway almost always follows wood pores. The arc is of fine diameter, typically a few millimeters in diameter, and indeed tends to "fine down" internally compared with externally. In the body, evidence of internal breakdown may similarly be found, as tissue planes are present, although of much broader dimension and therefore more current diffusing. There are other reasons why a path may not be found, however. The most likely medium for transmission is the vascular tree, with its ionic liquid content. If current is transmitted internally via this medium, post-mortem evidence may not be present. Even so, such conduction is likely to be quite dangerous, leading directly to the heart.

We now turn to an examination of likely current magnitudes and pathways. In light of the foregoing discussion, three cases are considered: (1) direct strike with no external flashover, (2) direct strike with external flashover, and (3) EPR shock. At least the first two cases are shown to engender shocks of lethal magnitude.

B. BODY MODEL

The model used for the body is shown in Figure 1. The components follow commonly accepted lines, and include a 1-kΩ internal resistance split between arms, torso, and legs as the internal component. This is purely resistive. The components for skin resistivity are significantly larger than for the internal resistance, and consist of a parallel resistance and capacitance

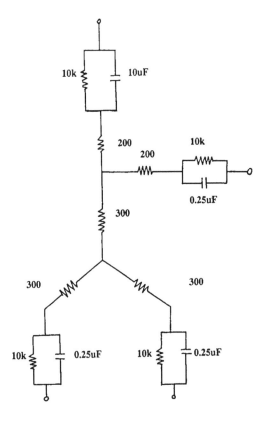

FIGURE 1. Body model.

of 10 kΩ and 0.25 μF, respectively. The skin is assumed to break down at a voltage of 5 kV across the parallel combination, and body surface breakdown to occur at a gradient of 2.7 kV/cm, or for a 1.8-m adult, approximately 500 kV. These are standard accepted values. Gaps G_1 to G_4 model the breakdown at various stages, with G_4 representing external flashover.

C. EARTH RESISTANCE COMPONENT

Meliopoulos[8] has derived expressions for earth resistance applicable to these conditions. For an individual standing on a surface of earth resistance ρΩ·m, the resistance measured from single foot to true earth is given by

$$R_e = \frac{\rho}{8b}$$

where ρ is the earth resistivity and b is the radius of the equivalent flat plate representing one foot. Thus, he shows that

$$R_e = 3\rho$$

approximately. In subsequent sections, ρ is taken to be 100 Ω·m.

D. DIRECT STRIKE

Two cases of direct strike are now considered. The first is assumed to be a direct strike with no external breakdown. An impulse of 5 kA using an 8/20-μs waveform is directly applied to the cranial skin, and the sequence of events shown in Figure 3 is observed using this model. The equivalent circuit is shown in Figure 2.

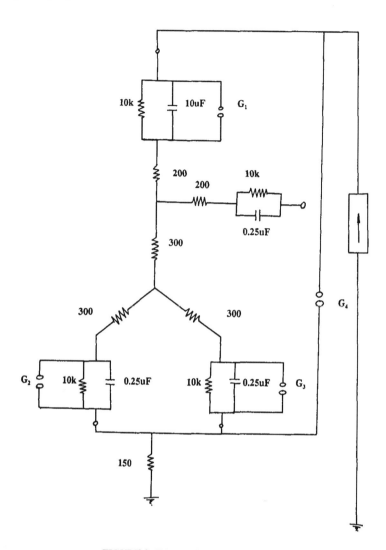

FIGURE 2. Direct strike equivalent circuit.

Even though no external flashover is modeled to occur in this example, skin breakdown is highly likely, and is programmed to occur at 5 kV. The sequence of events shows that:

1. Current rises exponentially in the internal milieux in pace, but lagging slightly behind the applied current. This is a capacitive effect.
2. At 1.1 and 1.7 µs, respectively, breakdown of skin components occurs. This only has marginal impact on the internal current.
3. Ultimately, a value of internal current in pace with the maximum value of the applied current is reached. This is 5 kA, and is an obviously harmful current.
4. By 100 µs, the current wave has largely decayed, and only a small component remains until 500 µs.

This situation is obviously harmful, and the degree of harm depends on the localization of the breakdown channel and the current density in the channel. It seems a reasonable worst-case assumption that this be conducted directly to the heart via the blood vessels, and probably is transmitted via the aorta, with a cross-sectional area of around 7 cm^2. The current density is thus extremely large.

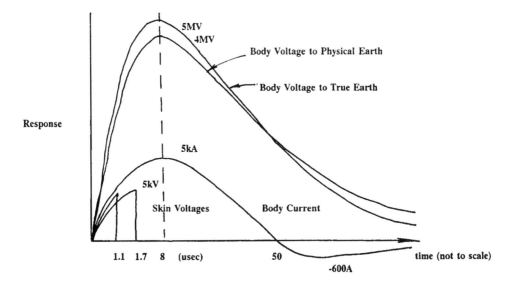

FIGURE 3. Time sequence of events. Direct strike, no flashover.

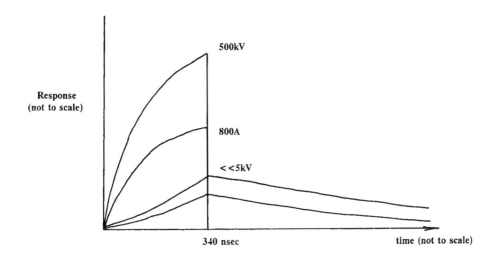

FIGURE 4. Time sequence of events. Direct strike, with flashover.

Dalziel's original work was not conducted at this brevity of impulse, but if we extrapolate as others have done, the lethal current at, say, 50 μs impulse duration is 16.4 A. Obviously, this is greatly exceeded and this circumstance is supremely dangerous.

The second case under consideration is that where the circumstances are as above, but external flashover occurs. The equivalent circuit is the same as the above, and the sequence of events is shown in Figure 4. The voltage between the cranium and local ground rises exponentially until 500 kV is reached, when external flashover occurs at approximately 340 ns after attachment. At this stage, the body current has risen to approximately 800 A. At flashover, the voltage and internal current drop dramatically to zero, and the vast majority of current is transmitted externally. The skin voltages now do not rise to 5 kV, and so electrical breakdown does not occur. It is highly likely, however, that mechanical disruption of the skin surface occurs, and so skin resistance markedly decreases. Nonetheless, the effect of this on body current is negligible.

Using Dalziel's criterion, the lethal current for a 340-ns impulse is 19.9 kA, and this is certainly exceeded. Thus, this circumstance also represents a highly dangerous situation.

It is stressed that Dalziel's criterion was not derived at such short impulse times. Others have extrapolated to this level, however (e.g., the Japanese group referred to above), and as the criterion is markedly exceeded, it serves simply as a guide to lethality. This guide is also supported by the recent IEC 479-1 and 2 reports for shorter-duration impulses.

E. HEATING CONSIDERATIONS

Other effects have been proposed for the effects of lightning damage to tissue, including heating effects. It is instructive to calculate possible temperature rises given the above possible scenarios.

The internal current rises to apporoximately 800 A in 340 ns, and if as a first approximation this is considered linear, the energy input is approximately 33 J. If this is dissipated in the heart with a volume of about 200 ml, and the specific heat of water, then the temperature rise is around 0.04°C. If, on the other hand, no flashover occurs, the current is much larger and the energy absorption is around 188 kJ, and the cardiac temperature rise would be potentially 224°C, which is obviously capable of producing thermal damage. Since damage of this magnitude is simply not seen, the worst-case assumption that this dissipation occurs totally within the myocardium is not valid.

The situation for metal on the body surface is significant, since it is claimed that heating of metal objects can cause contact burns. Indeed, this may be so, for if a piece of metal is in the path of a 5-kA flashover, and is perhaps a piece of jewelry with a resistance of 1 Ω, then the energy absorbed will be of the order of 625 J. If the metal weighs 100 g and is of material such as aluminum with a specific heat of 0.21 cal/g/°C, then the temperature rise will be 7°C. This is unlikely to cause thermal burns, though the metal may cause current concentrations and arcing to the skin beneath. This may explain the contact burns seen in the injury.

F. EPR-MEDIATED SHOCK

The remaining case for consideration is EPR-mediated shock. The equivalent circuit for this circumstance is shown in Figure 5. The equivalent circuit for the applied voltage is that given by Meliopoulos.[8] The magnitude of the voltage source is given by

$$V_{eq} = \frac{\rho I}{2\pi} \left\{ \frac{1}{r_1} - \frac{1}{r_2} \right\}$$

where r_1 and r_2 are the distances of the body parts in contact with physical ground from the base of the lightning stroke. The other quantities are defined as before. R_{eq} is given by 1.5ρ, being two 3-ρ resistances in parallel.

If we assume a 5-kA lightning stroke and a person 10 m distant with legs 1 m apart, V_{eq} is 800 V, and is thus approximated as 1 kV in the model. If the person is 20 m from the base of the stroke, then the voltage falls to 200 V, and it may be seen that EPR (in the field) is a relatively small effect.

When these parameters are introduced to the model, a current of approximately 1.05 A, peak, flows through the legs. Modeled in this way, the myocardium seems at no risk; however, it must be remembered that the internal resistance is distributed rather than discrete in reality. Thus, a small current will flow peripherally through the myocardium. The accepted factor applied due to a leg-to-leg current is less than 0.3, and so it is expected that less than 300 mA will flow. This is unlikely to be dangerous, on IEC and Dalziel criteria, given the small duration (45 µs) of the impulse. The effect for a large animal, e.g., cattle, with legs up to 4 m apart and direct transthoracic pathways, may well be less comforting.

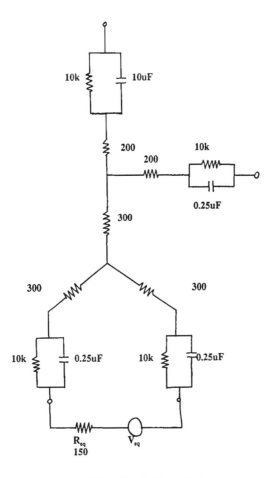

FIGURE 5. EPR-mediated strike equivalent circuit.

REFERENCES

1. **Blake-Pritchard, E. A.,** Changes in the central nervous system due to electrocution, *Lancet*, 1, 1163, 1934.
2. **Ishikawa, T., Ohashi, M., Kitigawa, N., Nagai, Y., and Miyazawa, T.,** Experimental study on the lethal threshold value of multiple successive voltage impulses to rabbits simulating multi-strike lightning flash, *Int. J. Biometeorol.*, 29(2), 157, 1985.
3. **Nagai, Y., Ishikawa, T., Ohashi, M., and Kitigawa, N.,** Study of lethal effects of multiple-stroke flash lethal effects on rabbits subjected to three successive voltage impulses simulating multiple-stroke flash (sic), *Res. Lett. Atm. Phys.*, 2, 87, 1982.
4. **Ishikawa, T., Miyazawa, T., Ohashi, M., et al.,** Experimental studies on the effect of artificial respiration after lightning accidents, *Res. Exp. Med. (Berl.)*, 179, 59, 1981.
5. **Ohashi, M., Kitigawa, N., and Ishikawa, T.,** Lightning injury caused by discharges accompanying flashovers — a clinical and experimental study of death and survival, *Burns*, 12(7), 496, 1986.
6. **Flisowski, Z. and Mazzetti, C.,** An approximate method of assessment of the electric shock hazard by lightning strike, *18th Int. Conf. Lightning Protection,* VDE-Verlag GMbH, 1985, 449 (paper 6.9).
7. **Darveniza, M.,** *Electrical Properties of Wood and Line Design,* University of Queensland Press, 1980.
8. **Meliopoulos, A. P.,** *Power System Grounding and Transients,* Marcel Dekker, New York, 1990.

II. CARDIORESPIRATORY SYSTEMS

C. J. Andrews

With the above discussion as background, we turn to the cardiovascular system and respiratory system with the expectation that most problems arise from either traumatic blast effects or direct effects of electric current on conduction characteristics of conducting tissues and membranes. And, indeed, this is largely what has been proposed.

Burda,[1] in noting diffuse T-wave inversion representing a pattern of generalized ischemia, proposes a diffuse myocardial electrical injury. Patchy myocardial necrosis with epicardial hemorrhage has been seen at post-mortem,[2,8] and also a generalized spiral myocardial muscle fibril malformation.[3] Similar findings have been seen in those subjected to direct current (DC) countershock (DCCS).[4] Contusion of the myocardium from "blast" is also postulated.[11]

Patterns of *localized* infarct on ECG are harder to explain. It has been proposed that coronary thrombosis forms secondary to vascular damage, precipitating infarct.[6] This has not been supported by post-mortem findings in lightning injury, and does not explain the resolution of these patterns as is the usual case. Thallium scan in such a patient has shown normal perfusion,[9] in the presence of transmural inferior changes.

Burda[1] has two alternative views. First, perhaps in the older patient, precipitation of an infarct in the already-compromised patient may occur. Second, with the centrally mediated respiratory arrest[6] and evolving hypoxia, myocardial anoxia may occur, and this coupled with a metabolic (possibly centrally mediated) hypersympathetic state may compromise the myocardium.[7]

This again does not explain focal patterns, and as an alternate view it may simply be that different current paths depending on different sites of the strike cause different current densities around the myocardium.

Alternatively, widespread T-wave changes are also seen in cerebral injuries,[7] a mechanism quite apropos of the lightning case.

Arrhythmia generation is easily explained by irritable damaged and hypoxic myocardial tissue. This is a standard mechanism. Electrical discharge of a degree more minor than lightning occurring in the late T-wave is known to be arrhythmogenic also, particularly of ventricular fibrillation. Ventricular fibrillation is now more often recognized than the classically reported asystole. The initial cardiac arrest is thought to be due to massive myocardial depolarization,[5] and is said to be profound systole followed by asystole. The effect, however, is local, as opposed to that of respiratory arrest, which is thought to be central.[5] There may however be a strong central vagal stimulation.[2]

Respiratory injury is seen in two forms. First, the initial respiratory arrest is thought to be central medullary in origin.[6,10] Second, blast contusion is seen.[12]

There is debate on whether the phenomenon of keraunoparalysis is vascular, neural, or neurohumoral in origin. ten Duis discusses it elsewhere in this volume.

REFERENCES

1. **Burda, C. A.,** Electrocardiographic changes in lightning stroke, *Am. Heart. J.*, 82 (521), 1966.
2. **Lynch, M. and Shorthouse, P. H.,** Injuries and death from lightning, *Lancet*, 1, 473, 1949.
3. **Jellinek, S.,** Death by lightning (letter), *Br. Med. J.*, December 12, 714, 1942.
4. **Tedeschi, C. G. and White, C. W., Jr.,** A morphological study of canine hearts subjected to fibrillation, electrical defibrillation, and manual compression, *Circulation*, 9, 916, 1954.
5. **Ravitch, M. M., Lane, R., Safar, P., Steichen, F., and Knowles, P.,** Lightning stroke, *N. Engl. J. Med.*, 264(1), 36, 1961.

6. **Imboden, L. E. and Newton, C. B.,** Myocardial infarction following electric shock, *U.S. Armed Forces Med. J.,* 3(3), 497, 1952.
7. **Chia, B. L.,** Electrocardiographic abnormalities and congestive cardiac failure due to lightning stroke, *Cardiology,* 68, 49, 1981.
8. **Subramanian, N.,** Cardiac injury due to lightning — report of a survivor, *Indian Heart J.,* 37(1), 72, 1985.
9. **Jackson, S. H. D.,** Lightning and the heart, *Br. Heart. J.,* 43, 454, 1980.
10. **Krob, M. J. and Kram, A. E.,** Lightning injuries: a multisystem trauma, *J. Iowa Med. Soc.,* 73(6), 221, 1983.
11. **Craig, S. R.,** When lightning strikes, pathophysiology and treatment of lightning injuries, *Postgrad. Med.,* 79(4), 109, 1986.
12. **Moulson, A. M.,** Blast injury of the lungs due to lightning, *Br. Med. J.,* 289, 1270, 1984.

III. PATHOPHYSIOLOGY OF LIGHTNING INJURY TO THE NERVOUS SYSTEM

M. J. Eadie

A. INTRODUCTION

Lightning-mediated injury to the human nervous system appears to be a relatively uncommon event. Its occurrence is determined largely by chance, although it is more frequent in those who are often involved in outdoor activities, either occupational or recreational. However, anyone happening to be outdoors in a thunderstorm is at an increased risk. Being inside buildings or other shelter does not provide complete protection. Contemporary knowledge of the pathophysiology of lightning injury to the nervous system has been derived from a retrospective analysis of the clinical and pathological features of such events in humans, and from analogy to the effects of accidental or punitive (i.e., legal) electrocution. There has been great difficulty in simulating the full extent of the lightning discharge in the research laboratory. However, it is possible to produce either high-voltage or high-current impulses, and these have been used for limited experimental study of the phenomena in animal models.

Because of the way in which we have derived our knowledge of the mechanisms of lightning injury to the nervous system, it seems sensible to consider the means by which the high-impulse current of lightning comes to have an effect on the body and the nervous system, and the mechanisms by which such current spreads through and injures the nervous system, before proceeding to discuss the actual recorded effects of lightning on the human nervous system.

B. MEANS WHEREBY LIGHTNING MAY AFFECT THE NERVOUS SYSTEM

There are several known means whereby lightning may impose its effects on the structure and/or functions of the nervous system. These means can be seen to fall into two main categories: (1) direct electrical ones and (2) indirect (nonelectrical) ones.

1. Direct Electrical Effects

Analysis of the relevant literature suggests that the direct electrical effects of lightning on the human body and nervous system may come about via three main mechanisms:

1. Direct lightning strike on the body
2. (Lateral) lightning "splash" onto the body after a direct lightning strike on a nearby object or person
3. Spread through the ground of an electrical potential (a "ground current") following the nearby earthing of a lightning discharge

Direct lightning strike — Lightning may achieve a direct strike on a human body, passing to earth through that body and over its surface. The point of the initial strike will almost always be that part of the body which projects furthest above the ground. Thus, in most instances, the human head will be struck, unless the victim is lying down or is in some unusual posture, or part of the body is in contact with some conducting material, e.g., metal jewelry, a metal-framed umbrella, or a golf club held in the hand. In the latter cases, the lightning is likely to make its initial strike on the conductor and then discharge into the body via the part in contact with the conductor. If this happens, the initial effect of the lightning on a neural structure may be on a portion of the peripheral nervous system. However, the usual effect of a lightning strike on the head of an upright human body will result in the current of the discharge having an initial effect on the underlying brain itself.

Lightning splash — If the lightning strike initially attaches to an object which is itself a relatively poor conductor, e.g., a tree, the discharge may jump laterally and may make a secondary contact with the nearest point of a human body close at hand. Alternatively, the lightning splash current may make secondary contact with a conductor which is in contact with part of the body and thence spread through the body to earth. The point of lightning contact will determine the initial site at which the discharge affects the nervous system.

Ground current (step voltage) — A lightning discharge which first strikes the earth may then spread laterally through the nearby ground, reach a human body in contact with that ground, and then enter that body. Commonly, the victim in this situation is standing with legs apart. When the ground current passes under the victim's legs, it induces a potential difference between the two legs (a stride potential). This results in the passage of current through the legs and lower trunk. With such a stride potential, the electrical effects of lightning are particularly likely to involve neural structures in the lower limbs and trunk.

C. CONSEQUENTIAL EFFECTS

There appear to be two main means whereby lightning may have consequential effects on the nervous system: (1) by producing cardiorespiratory arrest and (2) via various mechanical consequences of the lightning strike.

1. Cardiorespiratory Arrest

Lightning strike may cause immediate cardiorespiratory arrest. The massive current involved in a lightning strike may cause profound myocardial depolarization and asystole as it spreads through the body.[1,2] It has also been suggested that the lightning current may depolarize the vagal nuclei in the medulla oblongata[3] and thus cause cessation of cardiac and respiratory activity through neurogenic mechanisms. The consequent cerebral ischemia may damage the nervous system.

2. Mechanical Effects

The bodies of those struck by lightning may be physically displaced from the positions they occupied at the moment of the strike. Several possible mechanisms have been invoked. Thus, it has been suggested[4] that the spread of lightning current through the body may cause massive contraction of the victim's skeletal muscle, of such power that his or her body is thrown from its original position.[5,6] Such tetanic contraction is more likely to occur with the continuing passage of the alternating current that occurs in electrocution than with the single, momentary direct-current surge that occurs in lightning injury. Another possibility is that the heat produced from a nearby lightning strike may set up a blast effect, and the resulting pressure wave may suddenly displace the bodies of persons and other movable objects in the vicinity,[2,7] thus causing

injury. These are the most probable explanations for the physical displacement of the bodies of lightning strike victims over appreciable distances. An earlier explanation lies in repulsion between induced like electrical charges,[8] but this has been largely discounted.[9]

The displacement of the victim's body produced by a nearby lightning strike may cause physical injury. This injury may happen to involve the central or peripheral nervous system by virtue of the various established mechanisms whereby physical injury may damage these structures.

It seems conceivable that lightning may affect a given individual by more than one of these injury mechanisms simultaneously. Thus, a lightning strike on a tree a short distance from a victim may cause nervous system injury both by direct lightning splash from the site of the primary strike and through bodily displacement effects, leading to head injury followed by, for instance, intracranial bleeding.

D. MECHANISMS THROUGH WHICH LIGHTNING DIRECTLY DAMAGES THE NERVOUS SYSTEM

As mentioned earlier, the postulated mechanisms whereby the electric current of a lightning strike causes direct damage to nervous tissue elements have not been established by experiment. Rather, they have been inferred from a number of items of evidence. It is possible that more than one of the inferred mechanisms may operate simultaneously in the one affected individual.

When an electric current enters the body, it moves toward earth preferentially along the most direct path of the lowest electrical resistance. The pulse of current engendered by the very high potential of a lightning discharge is likely to earth itself by spread over the body surface, particularly if there is a superficial layer of sweat or moisture, and also by spread through the body tissues in a direct path between point of contact and earth. The circulating blood, with its ionic content of plasma, the CSF, and the muscle mass constitute the preferential pathways of current movement toward earth within the body. The literature seems to contain little discussion as to whether the lightning current will also spread along neural structures, although one might anticipate that the sudden direct-current surge would depolarize them.

A lightning current surge through the body might be expected to damage neural structures by at least two possible mechanisms: (1) local heating and (2) induced ionization of tissue molecules. More than 50 years ago, Blake-Pritchard[8] published a set of calculations, primarily in relation to the effects of electrocution on the nervous system, but also taking into account the mechanisms of lightning injury. He estimated that, in legal electrocution, the heating effect of the electrical current could raise the temperature of the CSF by 33°C. He was unable to derive a corresponding figure for a lightning current, although the higher voltages involved suggested that the temperature rise in CSF and blood might be even greater. Blake-Pritchard[8] considered that the temperature rise due to the current would not suffice to cause the CSF or blood to boil, or to expand sufficiently to damage tissues through mechanical effects. However, probably because of the state of contemporary knowledge, he did not consider the consequences of the hyperthermia on the rate of biochemical reactions or on tissue ultrastructure. As to ionization produced by the electrical current, he believed that the total electrical energy of a typical lightning flash (some 20 C) would be capable of ionizing sufficient H_2O molecules in the body to liberate only 1 ml of oxygen and 2 ml of hydrogen. Such volumes of gas would be expected to have trivial mechanical consequences on the structure of body tissues. Again, he paid no attention to the possible disruptive effect of induced molecular ionization on biochemical reactions. Blake-Pritchard[8] did not proceed to develop a quantitative argument in connection with the effects of lightning in inducing electrostatic charges in body tissues. However, in part by virtue of his belief that neither the heating nor the ionizing effect of lightning was adequate to explain the observed tissue damage, he took the view that electrostatic changes were the main cause of tissue injury. He did calculate that lightning would induce charges on the victim, and on nearby objects, that would be of a magnitude sufficient to explain the distances over which victims' bodies were displaced in lightning accidents. By analogy, he seemed to infer that similar repulsions between induced like charges would occur within the victim's body and that these would produce distortions and displacements of tissue elements. Bearing in mind the ionic nature of the internal environment of the body, the brevity of the lightning current, the known "pinch-in" behavior of arcs,[7] and the elastic properties of many body tissues, one questions the validity of this particular line of argument.

Over the half century since Blake-Pritchard's work, additional evidence has come to light which may help explain the mechanisms through which lightning damages the nervous system. There has first been the realization that the effect of lightning on the myocardium is akin to that of a direct-current countershock in causing massive myocardial depolarization, with asystole. Conceivably, a similar effect occurs in other excitable tissue, including the nervous system, so that a lightning discharge may cause local or widespread suppression of neural activity by a direct electrical effect. Second, when a lightning victim is affected by a stride potential, there is commonly a phase where the lower limbs are pulseless and ischemic.[10] This phase is usually temporary, but may last for many minutes or longer. The syndrome has sometimes been ascribed to the consequences of a massive autonomic discharge activated by the lightning current as it spreads through the victim's trunk.[11] This may be so, but the possibility arises that the lightning current passage along and within arteries in the lower limbs may cause arterial wall contraction and thus vasospasm. Further, there may be local heating of endothelium which may contribute to, or be responsible for, local thrombosis and diminished peripheral blood flow. Reports of arterial thrombosis in limbs affected by high-voltage electrical discharges[12] suggest that direct arterial wall injury may at least at times be a relevant possibility. Similar arterial injury may lead to ischemic damage to the neural structures these vessels supply. Arterial spasm, with later thrombosis at sites of endothelial injury, could explain the development of evidence of damage at a relevant level of the nervous system which appears hours to days after a lightning injury (see, e.g., Reference 13).

There is no reason why more than one of these various pathogenic mechanisms may not apply in a given individual in causing nervous system damage after a lightning strike. An understanding of these possibilities helps in interpreting the neuropathology and clinical features of lightning injury to the nervous system.

E. NEUROPATHOLOGY

The literature contains a number of descriptions of the neuropathological changes associated with lightning injury.[8,14-16] Unfortunately, in some of the descriptions, lightning injuries have not been sharply differentiated from consequences of electrocution.

1. Entry- and Exit-Site Injuries

There is often a pattern of skin burns at, and radiating from, the point of lightning entry into the body. Sometimes there is more extensive tissue injury, perhaps amounting to ulceration, at the points of current entry and exit.

2. Central Nervous System

Necropsy material from lightning victims has often been reported to show brain congestion with widespread petechial hemorrhages over the cerebral surface, particularly beneath the current entry point. Not infrequently, there is some subarachnoid bleeding. Foci of petechial hemorrhage may occur throughout the parenchyma of the cerebral hemispheres and basal ganglia, the midbrain, the medulla, hypothalamus, and the spinal cord. Sometimes there are large vascular tears and rents within the cerebrum.[14] The vascular tears may provide the pathological correlate of the intracerebral hematomas noted on CT head scanning in recent years in survivors of lightning strike.[17] The CSF spaces, both those over the cerebral hemispheres and the Virchow-Robin spaces, have often been described as dilated,[8,14] and there has been separation of adjacent neocortical layers. In contrast, some descriptions have mentioned the presence of edema of the whole brain[18] or of the subcortical white matter.[15,16] In severe injuries the whole brain and spinal cord may be softened.[14] However, at post-mortem, the brains of some lightning victims have shown no edema.[15] Neurons often show microscopic abnormalities. Critchley[14] reported chromatolysis of pyramidal, medullary, and anterior horn neurons and Purkinje cells, while Blake-Pritchard[8] spoke of ganglion cell damage. Lynch and Shorthouse[15] pointed out that the distribution of chromatolytic neurons in the lightning-injured brain was patchy, affected and intact neurons sometimes lying within 100 to 200 μm of each other. The cerebral blood vessels may also be injured. Blake-Pritchard[8] described rupture of the muscular coats of these vessels.

It is difficult to assess the extent to which cerebral hypoxia from circulatory arrest may have contributed to certain of the described neuropathological abnormalities, but clearly the totality of structural changes amounts to more than the effects of hypoxia alone. In particular, the tears in the cerebral substance, and the clustering of small hemorrhages beneath the site of lightning entry, appear to be likely consequences of electrical trauma itself. The dilated perivascular spaces seem to have an unusual appearance, but one which has been remarked on in several reports. According to Lynch and Shorthouse,[15] this dilatation has been ascribed to the effects of heating or to electrolytic liberation of gas. The possibility does not seem to have been mentioned that the dilatation might be a fixation or embedding artifact resulting from altered neural parenchymal consistency, itself a consequence of the passage of the lightning current.

3. Peripheral Nerves

Critchley[14] described "striking localized ballooning" of the myelin sheaths of peripheral nerves in cases of severe electrical injury, but it is not clear whether this change also occurred in cases of lightning injury.

REFERENCES

1. **Cooper, M. A.,** Lightning injuries: prognostic signs for death, *Ann. Emerg. Med.,* 9, 134, 1980.
2. **Craig, S. R.,** When lightning strikes. Pathophysiology and treatment of lightning injuries, *Postgrad. Med.,* 79, 109, 1986.
3. **Alexander, L.,** Clinical and neuropathological aspects of electrical injuries, *J. Ind. Hyg. Toxicol.,* 20, 191, 1938.
4. **Strasser, E. J., Davis, R. M., and Manchey, M. J.,** Lightning injuries, *J. Trauma,* 17, 315, 1977.
5. **Apfelberg, D. B., Masters, F. W., and Robinson, D. W.,** Pathophysiology and treatment of lightning injuries., *J. Trauma,* 14, 453, 1974.
6. **Peters, W. J.,** Lightning injury, *Can. Med Assoc. J.,* 128, 148, 1983.
7. **Darveniza, M.,** Electrical aspects of lightning injury and damage, in *Lightning Injuries: Electrical, Medical, and Legal Aspects,* Andrews, C. J., Cooper, M. A., Darveniza, M., and Mackerras, D., Eds., CRC Press, Boca Raton, FL, 1992, chap. 3.
8. **Blake-Pritchard, E. A.,** Changes in the central nervous system due to electrocution, *Lancet,* 1, 1163, 1934.
9. **Golde, R. H. and Lee, W. R.,** Death by lightning, *Proc. Inst. Electr. Eng.,* 123, 1163, 1976.
10. **ten Duis, H.,** Keraunoparalysis, in *Medical Aspects of Lightning Injury,* Andrews, C. J., Cooper, M. A., Darveniza, M., and Mackerras, D., Eds., CRC Press, Boca Raton, FL, 1991, chap. 6, sect. IV.
11. **Sharma, M. and Smith, A.,** Paraplegia as a result of lightning injury, *Br. Med. J.,* 2, 1464, 1978.
12. **Hunt, J. L., McManus, W. F., Haney, W. P., and Pruitt, B. A., Jr.,** Vascular lesions in acute electrical injuries, *J. Trauma,* 14, 461, 1974.
13. **Langworthy, O. R.,** Abnormalities produced in the central nervous system by electrical injuries, *J. Exp. Med.,* 51, 943, 1930.

14. **Critchley, M.,** Neurological effects of lightning and of electricity, *Lancet,* 1, 68, 1934.
15. **Lynch, M. J. G. and Shorthouse, P. H.,** Injuries and death from lightning, *Lancet,* 1, 473, 1949.
16. **Panse, F.,** Electrical trauma, in *Handbook of Clinical Neurology,* Vol. 23, Vinken, P. J. and Bruyn, G. W., Eds., North-Holland, Amsterdam, 1975, 683.
17. **Stanley, L. D. and Suss, R. A.,** Intracerebral hematoma secondary to lightning stroke: case report and review of the literature, *Neurosurgery,* 16, 686, 1985.
18. **Kotagal, S., Rawlings, C. A., Chen, S., Burria, G., and Nouri, S.,** Neurologic, psychiatric, and cardiovascular complications in children struck by lightning, *Pediatrics,* 70, 190, 1982.

IV. KERAUNOPARALYSIS

H. J. ten Duis

Temporary paralysis of one or more extremities following a lightning strike is called keraunoparalysis or Charcot's paralysis. This acute neurological disorder can be induced by all known basic mechanisms by which lightning can affect a person.

Reviewing the historical literature, case reports describing "lightning" paralysis can be found from the beginning of the nineteenth century.[1] A detailed description of the syndrome has been given by Boudin,[2] Duchenne,[3] Nothnagel,[4] and Charcot.[5]

The clinical symptoms of keraunoparalysis include flaccid paralysis of the extremities involved, mostly the legs, in combination with complete or partial sensory loss. In many cases there are signs of disturbed peripheral circulation: loss of pulse, extreme coolness, and a pale or livid blue discoloration of the skin.[6-9] As a rule, paralysis, sensory loss, and circulation disturbances disappear completely within 12 to 24 h, and in the majority of cases, even within 1 h. This means that clinical observation of the syndrome is seldom possible. The return of the peripheral circulation parallels the resolution of the neurological disorders; it is often accompanied by a tingling sensation or ischemic pain.

Many authors have tried to give a pathophysiological explanation for the phenomena observed. In general, they are ascribed to a motor, sensory, and vasomotor peripheral nerve reaction to the high current flow through the affected limb (see References 4, 5, and 7). Critchley[10] and Currens[11] believed the flaccid paralysis and sensory disturbances to be secondary to impaired peripheral circulation, because return of sensibility and muscle activity seemed to be directly related to restoration of the peripheral limb circulation. However, it is also possible that the activating mechanism works in just the opposite manner, because in some cases[1,7] paralysis has been observed without the complete loss of arterial circulation which is needed to provoke the actual neurological disturbances. Extreme vasoconstriction in the myelum was brought forward by Panse as an explanation for the clinical picture.[12] The observation of paralysis in patients in whom the entry and exit points of the current were located on the same extremity, without the myelum being interconnected in the electrical pathway, contradict this opinion.[13]

The induction of keraunoparalysis is independent of the direction of current flow, i.e., from central to peripheral or vice versa. When both arms or both legs are connected in series, keraunoparalysis can be observed in adjacent limbs where an afferent and subsequently an efferent current has flowed, thus being independent of the direction in which the lightning current has traversed the extremity. A good example is a lightning victim who has suffered exposure to a high stride potential. If the legs are some distance apart, part of the current traveling through the ground will flow up one leg and down the other.[6,8]

Comparable mechanisms have been described in patients in whom the upper and lower extremities were connected in series.[11] This can be observed in the case of a direct strike or side flash, when the current flows through an arm and then to ground through the legs and feet.

In theory, the vasomotor disturbances and stagnant arterial flow in the paralyzed extremities may result in muscle ischemia, subsequent anaerobic glycolysis and metabolic acidosis, and, consequently, in muscle cell injury. When recirculation has been established, secondary edema formation can be expected, so it may be necessary to perform fasciotomies. In practice, however, the usual, very transient nature of the symptoms of keraunoparalysis seldom necessitate extensive surgical therapy. The use of heparin has been advanced as a means of preventing clotting after vascular stasis in the affected limbs. This is controversial and not supported by formal studies. Indeed, heparin in the context of other trauma is used only with great caution. Infusion of colloid solutions with a proven antisludge activity may be a safer and equally effective modality. The treatment of keraunoparalysis remains controversial and, indeed, its transient nature makes treatment rarely necessary.

REFERENCES

1. **Stricker, W.,** Die Wirkung des Blitzes auf den Menschlichen Korper, in *Archiv fur pathologische Anatomie und Physiologie und fur klinische Medicin,* Bd. XX, Virchow, R., Ed., Georg Reimer Verlag, Berlin, 1860, 45.
2. **Boudin, M.,** Histoire medicale de la foudre et de ses effects sur l'homme, les animaux, les plantes, les edifices, les navires, *Ann. Hyg. Publique Med. Leg. II,* Ser. T II, 395; T III, 241; T IV, 241, 1854-55.
3. **Duchenne, G. B.,** *L'Electrisation Localisee,* 2nd ed., J. B. Bailliere et Fils, Paris, 1861.
4. **Nothnagel, H.,** Zur Lehre von der Wirkungen des Blitzes auf den thierischen Korper, *Virchow's Arch.,* 80, 327, 1880.
5. **Charcot, J. M.,** Wirkung des Blitzschlages auf das Nervensystem, *Wien. Med. Wochenschr.,* 40, 10, 1890.
6. **ten Duis, H. J., Klasen, H. J., and Reenalda, P. E.,** Keraunoparalysis, a "specific" lightning injury, *Burns,* 12, 54, 1985.
7. **Gathier, J. C.,** Neurological changes in a soldier struck by lightning, *Psychiatr. Neurol. Neurochir.,* 63, 125, 1960.
8. **Golde, R. H. and Lee, W. R.,** Death by lightning, *Inst. Electr. Eng. Rev.,* 123, 1163, 1976.
9. **Strasser, E. J., Davis, R. M., and Menchey, M. J.,** Lightning injuries, *J. Trauma,* 17, 315, 1977.
10. **Critchley, M.,** Injuries from electricity and lightning, *Br. Med. J.,* 1, 1217, 1935.
11. **Currens, J. H.,** Arterial spasm and transient paralysis resulting from lightning striking an airplane, *J. Aviat. Med.,* 16, 275, 1945.
12. **Panse, F.,** Die Neurologie des electrischen Unfalls und des Blitzschlages, in *Klinische Elektropathologie,* Arbeit u. Gesundheit Sozial. Med. Schriftenreihe a.d. Geb. des Bundesminist. für Arbeit, Heft 55, Koeppen, S. and Panse, F., Eds., Thieme Verlag, Stuttgart, 1955.
13. **Keller,** Falle von Blitzverletzung, *Dtsch. Med. Wochenschr.,* 39, 1233, 1917.

V. PSYCHOPATHOLOGY

B. Raphael and R. Cash

The thought of being struck by lightning is appalling to most people, with implications of instant death, of "being fried", of somehow being picked out for death by an "Act of God" or "Fate", or of being punished or chosen. Such powerful psychological themes surround all such experiences and must influence both the reactions of those so affected and the perceptions of the experience by those otherwise involved.

There are almost no systematic studies on the psychiatric sequelae of lightning stroke. There are a number of case reports from which a reasonable idea of such sequelae can be gleaned.

A. EFFECTS ON THE VICTIM

When lightning strikes a person, particularly, though not exclusively, if it strikes the person on the head, temporary or permanent cerebral damage is often the result. The person struck is often immediately rendered unconscious (see Chapter 5). Victims who have some return to consciousness usually recover and are highly unlikely to die.[1]

During the recovery period, the patient often becomes delirious. In 1890, Charcot[2] described what he called "the delirium of the man struck by lightning": pallor, trembling, disorientation of thought and confusion of speech, repetitiveness, and emotional lability. An illustrative case example is provided by Moran et al.[3] A 10-year-old boy was hit by lightning while sheltering under a tree. He regained consciousness after 24 h, although he remained confused, disoriented, and amnesic. He had amnesia for the initial event and the subsequent 10 d. After discharge, at 18 d, he became withdrawn and irritable and developed personality changes.

One can obtain a rough idea of the diversity and the consistencies in the clinical picture, and of the frequency of psychiatric problems, by looking at the few studies where groups of people have been considered. Iranyi et al[4] recorded some details of the 106 survivors out of 156 lightning casualties recorded in Hungary from 1959 to 1960. Panse[5] noted that two thirds of the survivors suffered impairment of consciousness lasting from a few minutes to several days. In a third of the cases with loss of consciousness, this was not followed by any lasting mental changes. In another third, the impairment of consciousness was followed by mental changes, with dullness, a sense of oppression, disorientation, a slowing of reaction times, and rarely, withdrawal and negativism. In eight cases, the disorder of consciousness fluctuated. In a few severe cases, psychosis of the "exogenous reaction type" developed, sometimes with delirium. This was sometimes accompanied by a state of agitation. One patient had to be transferred to a mental hospital. Seven of the victims who had suffered no prior loss of consciousness presented transient mental symptoms in the form of feelings of oppression, emotional lability, or narrowing of consciousness.

Panse also reports on a group of 29 people affected by a single lightning stroke. Three people were killed and 26 sustained some degree of injury. Fourteen of the victims were given neurological and psychiatric examinations 10 d after the trauma, and seven others provided useful reports on themselves. None of the 21 had been struck on the head. There was a high degree of similarity in the clinical picture and its course. Typically, there was some degree of clouding of consciousness, transient disturbance of motor and sensory functions of single or multiple limbs, autonomic nervous disorders, and what Panse describes as psychological and psychiatric reactions according to the underlying personality of the victim.

Arden et al[6] reported on an incident when lightning struck a tea stall at the Ascot Raceway, throwing a considerable number of people near the stall to the ground. Many of the patients admitted to the hospital had neurological signs and symptoms. Arden noted that in a few cases paresthesia persisted for several weeks, and in one case this was associated with "an hysterical ataxic gait". Critchley[7] commented in 1932 that many at that time inclined to the view that the paralytic symptoms of lightning stroke victims were psychogenic in type. In support of this idea, he emphasized the abrupt onset of symptoms after a dramatic and catastrophic cataclysm and the transient nature of the symptoms. In Critchley's much-quoted 1934 article,[8] he states that hysterical manifestations are very common after lightning stroke, that a great many cases of blindness, deafness, and loss of speech are on record, and that psychogenic symptoms are likely.

Although it is undoubtedly true that anxiety can sensibly be cited to explain some symptoms reported in post-lightning-stroke patients, the term "hysterical" and the psychological mechanisms implied by that term have faded from the literature over the past few decades.

Arden et al.[6] note that most of the patients from the Ascot incident had no residual symptoms, but that a few had emotional disturbances. We are given no details about what kind of emotional disturbances these few patients had. It is probable that Arden et al. were referring to the emotional lability and mood disturbances described above that are often a part of the organic brain syndrome in patients recovering from lightning stroke.

Kotagal et al.[9] have recorded the case of an 11-year-old boy struck by lightning while playing soccer. Soon after the accident, he was confused and disoriented. Three weeks following the accident, he developed frequent eqisodes of denial of the accident, marked agitation, and crying. He became emotionally labile and often expressed a fear of dying. He was often depressed. These disturbances of mood and behavior gradually resolved over the ensuing months with supportive psychotherapy. EEGs within the first and fourth weeks after the accident showed a generalized slowing in the 5 to 6-Hz range during wakefulness. A CT scan was normal.

The early confusion, disorientation, and memory problems are surely part of a delirium induced by the effects of the lightning on cerebral functioning. The latter symptoms can easily be understood in psychological terms, but the abnormal EEG in the fourth week after the accident, 1 week after these symptoms first appeared, leads to a presumption that organic factors also played a major role in the production of these symptoms.

Such EEG phenomena are also present in other reports where psychiatric symptoms are noted. Apfelberg et al.[10] described a case of a 68-year-old man who was struck by lightning while driving a tractor. Following an initially relatively uneventful recovery, at 4 months he was noted to have slurred speech, slow reaction, progressive weakness, clumsy movements of the right arm, and a tremor. He also had very labile emotions and deep depression. EEG showed diffuse, slow wave activity.

When reading such case histories in the literature, it is often impossible to decide whether organic or psychological factors are the predominant factors leading to the symptoms noted. Speculation on the issue is fruitless and detrimental if it reinforces an either/or approach to thinking about causality, which is inappropriate in these as in many instances in psychiatry.

When looking for psychological explanations for some of the symptoms following lightning stroke, the lack of well-designed research studies is even more apparent. Again one can speculate based on some of the symptoms reported in individual case histories. It seems sensible and not pushing speculation too far to propose that such a cataclysmic and overwhelming event as being struck by lightning could lead to post-traumatic stress disorder.

Another of Kotagal et al.[9]'s 11-year-old soccer players continued to have frequent episodes of depression, emotional lability, and impaired concentration on schoolwork for some time after the accident. He had recurrent thoughts pertaining to the accident for approximately 3 months, followed by a spontaneous resolution. Myers et al.[11] reported on a lightning strike which involved 47 children. One 15-year-old girl who had quite serious injuries had recurrent fear reactions for several days after the accident.

The recurrent thoughts pertaining to the accident reported by Kotagal et al.[9] in the 11-year-old soccer player and the recurrent fear reactions reported in the 15-year-old girl by Myers et al.[11] suggest anxiety and post-traumatic stress reactions. Panse[12] described a strange calm and lack of interest in several people from a group of 29 victims of a single lightning stroke. Such a numbing of responsiveness forms part of the current concept of post-traumatic stress disorder. Critchley[7] quotes case histories, some from the nineteenth century, of what he calls "psycho-recidivies", i.e., patients whose former psychological and somatic symptoms reappear with each succeeding thunderstorm.

The only attempt to examine, in any systematic way, anxiety-based sequelae in lightning stroke victims was by Dollinger[13, 14] and colleagues. In attempting to understand the development of psychiatric symptomatology following a lightning stroke, Dollinger's studies are unique in the literature and warrant detailed examination.

Dollinger et al.[13] investigated fears in children whose soccer game was interrupted by a lightning bolt that killed one child and injured several others. They compared the fears reported by these children with matched control children. Thirty-eight children from 35 families, the majority aged 10 to 12 years, took part in the study.

Based on an interview with the children and one parent about 1 month after the accident, and on behavioral observations taken during that interview, plus information from a 9-month follow-up, eight children were judged to be severly affected emotionally by the disaster. Three children had symptoms of generalized anxiety in many life situations. Another three boys were also extremely anxious, but their symptoms were much more focused, specifically on the possibility of stormy weather. At the mere sight of clouds or feeling of wind gusts, they would refuse to stay outdoors. They became upset when storms were forecast and were "petrified" during thunderstorms.

Seven boys were judged to be moderately affected, with problems similar to the above. Fifteen children were slightly affected and eight were judged to be relatively unaffected emotionally by the incident. Five children in the sample were reported to have some form of adjustment or learning problem prior to the incident. These five children were neither more nor less upset by the disaster than their counterparts.

The children were given a thematic apperception task. The stories told by the children suggested that the children's sense of subjective probability about lightning was dramatically increased—the "it can happen to me" phenomenon. Because there was a strong tendency to devise positive outcomes when the lightning inflicted some personal injury, Dollinger argued that this could reflect the children's efforts to obtain distance from the reality and impact of the event, perhaps through denial or repression. The author noted that such conclusions must necessarily be tentative, as there was no control group for this part of the research.

Explicit attribution of fear or anxiety to story characters correlated significantly with emotional upset in the child. Correlations were found between emotional upset and whether or not the sense of sight—looking at the lightning—was explicitly mentioned in the stories. Those children who did not mention sight were significantly more upset and more likely to have sleep disturbances and somatic complaints. Dollinger inferred from this that one mechanism used by the more upset children was a kind of selective inattention to some details. Two problems not found were hysterical manifestations and disaster-related games, such as those described by Terr.[15]

Dollinger et al.,[14] in another study on many of the same children, evaluated the respondent conditioning theory of the origin of children's fears by comparing the fears in the lightning stroke group to matched controls selected from a normative study. The theory proposes that a high-intensity stimulus can result in a conditioned fear and that this conditioned fear can generalize to other similar stimuli.

With mother-reported fears, only storm-related fears showed a significant difference between the lightning stroke and control groups. There was no fear generalization gradient. The child-reported fears did show, for the most part, the expected gradient. Storm fears showed the strongest magnitude. At a lesser magnitude were a number of other fears, most of which were conceptually related to the disaster in a meaningful way. Fears of sleep, noise, disaster, death, and bodily penetration were more prominent in the lightning stroke group.

The final expectation derived from learning theory is that stimuli unrelated to the traumatic incident should not show an elevated fearfulness. Consistent with this expectation, there were no group differences for obsessive fears or fears of school, embarrassment, or people.

There were some surprising results. In the intermediate range were increased fears of animals, supernatural events, and enclosed spaces which would seem to have little to do with the disaster. Dollinger et al.[14] suggested that from a psychodynamic perspective, these fears might represent displaced anxieties following the traumatic event, or regression to earlier forms of affective functioning. The authors argued that such a dynamic perspective should also lead to the expectation of an increased separation anxiety in the children. Significant separation anxiety failed to materialize for the sample as a whole. Thus, although displaced anxiety may have operated for some case histories, it was not prominent for most.

B. EFFECT ON OTHERS

While it is obvious that family members will be distressed if someone is struck by lightning and survives, it is clear that major problems will arise if the person is seriously injured or killed. The first author (B.R.) has treated bereaved persons following such deaths, and highly complicated and severe grief is a likely consequence. This is the more so because of the sudden, shocking, and unanticipated death that seems to have "chosen" one person, often someone young. It is often extremely difficult for families to come to terms with why an "Act of God" should have happened in this way.

C. CONCLUSIONS

There have been almost no studies devoted predominantly to examining the psychiatric sequelae in victims of lightning stroke. Although not as rare as many might think (see Chapter 4), being struck by lightning is still uncommon enough to ensure that most of the literature containing basic data consists of case reports, usually of a small number of cases which have come to a particular author's attention.

Despite this limitation, there are enough such reports for some confident conclusions to be drawn. Many people, including many rendered unconscious by the lightning stroke, recover without any psychiatric complications. A significant minority are delirious during the recovery period, with fluctuating levels of consciousness, attention and concentration, and memory deficits. Most, but not all, of this minority have affective changes as well, with mood lability, depression, or intense agitation being the most commonly reported problems.

Many of the somatic and psychic symptoms formerly thought to be hysterical in nature are no longer considered to be so.

While it is true that there are many reports of people left with permanent brain damage, it is also true that almost all who recover do so completely. There is EEG evidence to suggest that the organic brain syndrome can be quite long lasting.

In a very small group to patients, the symptoms gradually shade into longer-term problems, usually of a phobic or post-traumatic nature. Some also develop anxiety-based symptoms without any prior demonstrable organic brain damage, or with only the most transient changes in gross cerebral functioning immediately following the lightning stroke. Psychological theories satisfactorily explain the development of anxiety-based symptoms, and there is some evidence which supports these theories. Almost all of this small group who develop longer-lasting psychological symptoms also seem to recover completely over a period of some months.

It will be helpful if skilled psychiatric assessment of all such cases can lead to more systematic studies of these effects and optimal ways of managing them.

REFERENCES

1. **Cooper, M. A.,** Lightning injuries: prognostic signs for death, *Ann. Emerg. Med.,* 9, 134, 1980.
2. **Charcot, J. M.,** Des accidens nerveux provoques par la fondre 1890; as cited in Lynch, M. J. G. and Shorthouse, P. H., Injuries and death from lightning, *Lancet,* 1, 473, 1949.
3. **Moran, K. T., Jagan, N. T., and Munster, A. M.,** Lightning injury: physics, pathophysiology and clinical features, *Ir. Med. J.,* 79(5), 120, 1986.
4. **Iranyi, K., Iranyi, J., Orovecz, B., and Somogyi, E.,** Neuropsychiatrische Erscheinungen nach Blitzschlagunfallen, *Psychiatr. Neurol. Med. Psychol.,* 6, 310, 1964.
5. **Panse, F.,** Electrical trauma, in *Handbook of Clinical Neurology,* Vol. 23, Vinken, P. J. and Bruyn, G. W., Eds., Elsevier, Amsterdam, 1975, chap. 34.
6. **Arden, G. P., Harrison, S. H., Lister, J., and Maudsley, R. H.,** Lightning accident at Ascot, *Br. Med. J.,* June, 1450, 1956.
7. **Critchley, M.,** The effects of lightning: with especial reference to the nervous system, *Bristol Med. Chir. J.,* P. 285, 1932.
8. **Critchley, M.,** Neurological effects of electric shocks, *Lancet,* 1, 68, 1934.
9. **Kotagal, S., Rawlings, C. A., Chen, S., Burris, G., and Nouri, S.,** Neurologic, psychiatric, and cardiovascular complications in children struck by lightning, *Pediatrics,* 70, 190, 1982.
10. **Apfelberg, D. B., Frank, W. M., and Robinson, D. W.,** Pathophysiology and treatment of lightning injuries, *J. Trauma,* 14(6), 453, 1974.
11. **Myers, C. J., Colgan, M. T., and VanDyke, D. H.,** Lightning-strike disaster among children, *JAMA,* 238, 1045, 1977.
12. **Panse, F.,** 1925; as cited in **Lynch, M. J. G. and Shorthouse, P. H.,** Injuries and death from lightning, *Lancet,* 1, 473, 1949.
13. **Dollinger, S. J., O'Donnell, J. P., and Staley, A. A.,** Lightning-strike disaster: effects on children's fears and worries., *J. Consult. Clin. Psychol.,* 52, 1028, 1984.
14. **Dollinger, S. J.,** Lightning-strike disaster among children, *Br. J. Med. Psychol.,* 58, 375, 1985.
15. **Terr, L. C.,** Forbidden games: post-traumatic child's play, *J. Am. Acad. Child Psychiatry,* 20, 741, 1981.

VI. OCULAR SYSTEM

F. Fraunfelder and M. Meyer

A. PATHOPHYSIOLOGY OF LIGHTNING INJURY TO THE EYE

Electrical current causes damage to the eye in two ways: (1) thermal injury from generation of heat and (2) physiologic changes resulting from current passing through organs.

1.   Thermal Injury from Generation of Heat

On passing through the tissues, an electrical current is liable to destroy cells by both heat and electrolysis. A superficial electrical injury may heat the pigmented portion of the iris, inducing lens protein denaturation and typical mid-peripheral anterior subcapsular opacity.[1,2] Similarly, a deeper penetrating electrical current could produce thermal localization in the retinal pigment epithelium with secondary heating of the overlying retina because the melanin granules of the pigment epithelium and choroid would logically constitute the resistive obstacle to current flow.[3]

2.   Physiologic Changes from Current Passing Through the Eye

a.   *Factors Determining Effects of Lightning on the Eye*

There are six factors which determine the effect of lightning on the eye: type, intensity, strength and pathway of current, duration of contact, and resistance of the tissues.

Type of current — The effect of atmospheric (direct current) and technical (alternating current) electricity on the eye is virtually the same. Because of the cylindrical shock wave produced by lightning, ocular contusions may occur. Traumatic cataract, retinal detachment, and optic nerve injuries may be attributed to the massive direct-current shock.

Intensity (amperage) and strength (voltage) of current — The intensity of the current (amperage) is a measurement of how much energy courses through the body, and is determined by the type of current and high or low frequency (for alternating current). Voltage effect is determined by the power source (low tension, <1000 V; high tension, >1000 V), the duration of exposure to the power source, and the extent to which the patient is grounded at the time of lightning strike. The injurious effect of an electric current depends primarily on its intensity, i.e., the number of amperes. The magnitude of a lightning discharge is 12,000 to 200,000 A, while an average streak of lightning contains 50 to 100 million V.[4] The voltage and current peaks reached by lightning are seldom attained in high-voltage electrical injuries.[1] Cataracts, which are more common with lightning injury than with electrical injuries, may be due to a direct heat effect generated by the lightning flash[1] or to damage of the lens epithelium and capsule generated by the electrical current, which causes changes in the permeability of the lens.[5] This disruption of the osmotic barrier is then responsible for alterations in the lens proteins and metabolism.

Duration of contact — Lightning shock is usually very brief. The average duration of the lightning current passing through the body is 0.001 to 0.01 s.

Pathway of the current — The pathway of the current through the body is crucial, for current passing through the head is more likely to produce immediate death by involving the respiratory center or the heart.[6]

Resistance of the tissues — The resistance in an adult resides mainly in the skin and is between 1000 and 5000 Ω, but moist skin and wet footwear can reduce this to 300 Ω. The concept that electrical current will usually attempt to flow through the path of least resistance may not always be true; the path may be largely dependent on the voltage.[7] If the eye is interposed in the electric circuit, the areas of highest resistance will result in greater damage if contact with the current is long enough. As current meets resistance, its energy is converted to heat, which causes the tissue damage. The most vulnerable components of the posterior eye to electrical current are the retinal, choroidal, and optic nerve circulations. The low-resistance retina and optic nerve appear relatively immune to direct electrical current injury, and damage to these structures typically follows retinal and choroidal vascular occlusion or incompetence.

B. CLINICAL MANIFESTATIONS

Ocular symptoms correlate closely with the extent of the electrical burn to the eye or central nervous system.[8] Significant structural damage to the eyes and orbits is unusual, unless the site of current entry is close to the eye. Cataract is the most commonly reported ocular injury following a lightning strike. The closer the site of electrical injury to the eye, the greater the likelihood of cataract formation. Eyelid injuries range from mild erythematous reactions and edema to extensive coagulative lesions resulting in eyelid necrosis and loss of substance. In some instances, the conjunctiva is also irreparably damaged, and the anterior segment of the eye is disorganized. Electrical injuries to the posterior segment of the eye are uncommon. In general, the more superficial ocular tissues bear the brunt of most electrical injuries to the head.

1. Skin and Eyelids

Lid lesions caused by lightning may range from a typical partial-thickness burn to a more serious ulcerated necrotic lesion.[9] Skin and eyelid lesions are normally thermal injuries.

2. Conjunctiva and Cornea

In lightning injuries, the conjunctiva may become hyperemic, with ciliary injection and varying degrees of chemosis.[9,10] The cornea may develop punctate or striate opacities in the interstitial layers or may show generalized cloudiness.[11] In electrical injuries, opacities sometimes spread from the deeper layers to make the cornea totally opaque within a week, yet later subside. In severe cases, there may be corneal ulcers or extensive necrosis, with permanent scarring or perforation.

3. Pupils

Fixed and dilated pupils are well recognized following a lightning strike and do not necessarily suggest a bad prognosis.[12] When iridocyclitis occurs, it may be mild and transient or severe and recurrent.[13] Transient or permanent autonomic disturbances involving ocular function may occur rarely following a lightning injury. These disturbances may include mydriasis, anisocoria, Horner's syndrome, failure of accommodation, and loss of red reflex.[12,14,15]

4. Lens

Cataracts are the most frequently seen intraocular lesion in lightning victims. Cataracts caused by lightning were first described by St. Yves in 1722.[16] The earliest changes are usually manifested in the anterior subcapsular layer where fine vacuoles appear, and are replaced later by punctate and linear opacities which may form jagged patterns (Figures 1 and 2).[5,17,18] Opacities may also appear beneath the posterior capsule, especially after lightning injury. They are generally progressive, but may remain stationary or even regress. There is probably no single causative factor; changes have been attributed variously to thermal damage to the subcapsular epithelial cells and to the lens fibers, or to physiologic alteration of the permeability of the lens capsule.

Two types of cataracts are recognized after lightning injury. One type is due to a concussion and results in minute tears of the lens capsule. This ordinary traumatic cataract is usually seen shortly after the injury. The other type of cataract is more characteristic of an injury caused by lightning or high-tension current; however, both the anterior and posterior capsules are usually affected secondary to lightning.

Although cataracts usually appear as early as 4 weeks and as late as 24 months after injury, they can result immediately or as late as 11 years later.[18] They are usually unilateral on the side proximal to the point of contact, but the contralateral eye may also be involved.[19] Although the cataracts may fade and normal transparency will return to the lens, they are generally progressive. The pathogenesis of these lens changes is not completely known. One theory holds that the electrical current has a direct coagulative effect on the proteins of lens cells, while a direct heat effect has also been suggested as a factor in cataract formation secondary to lightning.

5. Posterior Segment

Lesions in the posterior segment are uncommon and usually due to physiologic changes. Vascular damages following lightning strikes may include narrowing of the arteries, dilatation of veins, hemorrhages, exudates, and edema.[20,21] The macula may undergo punctate pigmentary degeneration, cystic change, or hole formation following edema. Papilledema, choroidal rupture, and atrophy have also been described, as has optic neuritis followed by atrophy of variable amounts, with proportionate defects in the visual fields.[22]

6. CNS Involvement

Electrical injuries to the central nervous system may also cause physiologic changes, including ocular muscle palsies and nystagmus.[23] Decreased visual acuity or even blindness resulting from a variety of causes has also been observed.[14]

C. SUMMARY

Both thermal and physiologic changes resulting from lightning strikes may cause ocular

95

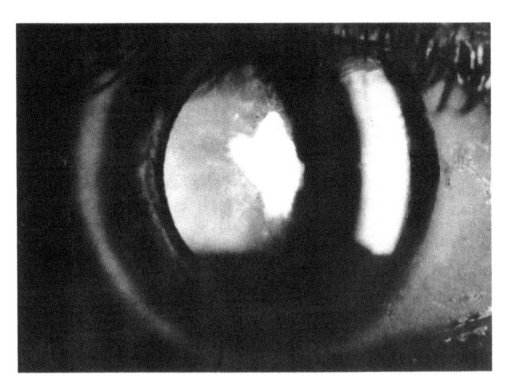

FIGURE 1. Slitlamp photograph of electrical cataract lens illustrating anterior position of central opacity. (From Hanna, C. and Fraunfelder, F. T., *Arch. Ophthalmol.*, 87, 18, 1972. With permission.)

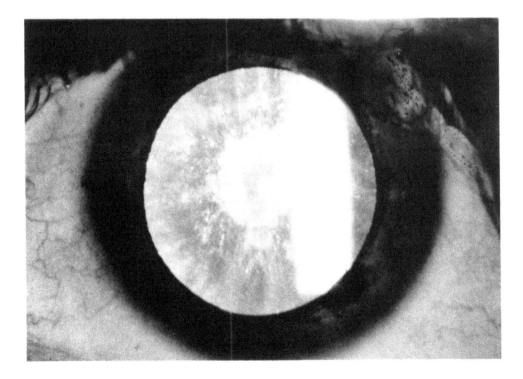

FIGURE 2. Slitlamp photograph of electrical cataract lens under retroillumination showing general orientation of fine opacities in anterior mid-periphery toward central cataract. (From Hanna, C. and Fraunfelder, F. T., *Arch. Ophthalmol.*, 87, 18, 1972. With permission.)

injuries. Cataracts are the most common ocular injury and usually appear 3 to 6 months after a lightning injury. Corneal damage secondary to lightning strikes generally consists of epithelial layer lesions which subside within weeks. Superficial thermal eyelid burns are also common, especially if the site of current entry was near the head.

REFERENCES

1. **Craig, S. R.,** When lightning strikes. Pathophysiology and treatment of lightning injuries, *Postgrad. Med.*, 79, 109, 1986.
2. **Hanna, C., Fraunfelder, F. T., and Johnston, G. C.,** Electrical induced cataracts, *Arch. Ophthalmol.*, 84, 232, 1970.
3. **Marmor, M. F. and Lurie, M.,** Light-induced electrical responses of the pigment epithelium, in *The Retinal Pigment Epithelium,* Zinn, K. and Marmor, M. F., Eds., Harvard University Press, Cambridge, 1978.
4. **Strasser, E. J., Davis, R. M., and Menchey, M. J.,** Lightning injuries, *J. Trauma,* 17, 315, 1977.
5. **Long, J. C.,** A clinical and experimental study of electric cataract, *Trans. Am. Ophthalmol. Soc.,* 60, 471, 1962.
6. **Solem, L., Fischer, R. P., and Strate, R. G.,** The natural history of electrical injury, *J. Trauma,* 17, 487, 1977.
7. **Hunt, J. L., Mason, A. D., Jr., Masterson, T. S., and Pruitt, B. A., Jr.,** The pathophysiology of acute electric injury, *J. Trauma,* 16, 335, 1976.
8. **Von Bahr, G.,** Electrical injuries, *Opthalmologica,* 158, 109, 1969.
9. **Noel, L.-P., Clarke, W. N., and Addison, D.,** Ocular complications of lightning, *J. Pediatr. Ophthalmol. Strabismus,* 17, 245, 1980.
10. **Peters, W. J.,** Lightning injury, *Can. Med. Assoc. J.,* 128, 148, 1983.
11. **Blake, J.,** Physical and chemical agents, in *Modern Ophthalmology,* Vol. 2, 2nd ed., Sorsby, A., Ed., Lippincott, Philadelphia, 1972, 622.
12. **Abt, J. L.,** The pupillary responses after being struck by lightning, *JAMA,* 254, 3312, 1985.
13. **Raymond, L. F.,** Specific treatment of uveitis, lightning induced: an auto-immune disease, *Ann. Allergy,* 27, 242, 1969.
14. **Castren, J. A. and Kytila, J.,** Eye symptoms caused by lightning, *Acta Ophthalmol.,* 42, 139, 1964.
15. **Lea, J. A.,** Paresis of accommodation following injury by lightning, *Br. J. Ophthalmol.,* 4, 417, 1920.
16. **Saint-Yves,** Nouveau traite des maladies des yeux, 368, 1722; as cited by Duke-Elder, S., *System of Ophthalmology,* Vol. 6, C. V. Mosby, St. Louis, 1954, 6435.
17. **Hanna, C. and Fraunfelder, F. T.,** Electric cataracts. II. Ultrastructural lens changes, *Arch. Ophthalmol.,* 87, 18, 1972.
18. **Fraunfelder, F. T. and Hanna, C.,** Electric cataracts. I. Sequential changes, unusual and prognostic findings, *Arch. Ophthalmol.,* 87, 179, 1972.
19. **Shapiro, M. B.,** Lightning cataracts, *Wis. Med. J.,* 83, 23, 1984.
20. **Moore, M. C.,** Ocular injury from lightning current and lightning flash, *Trans. Ophthalmol. Soc. Aust.,* 16, 87, 1956.
21. **Campo, R. V. and Lewis, R. S.,** Lightning-induced macular hole, *Am. J. Ophthalmol.,* 97, 792, 1984.
22. **Alexandridis, A., Fotiou, F., Dimitriadis, A., Tsitsopoulos, Ph., and Stefani, F. H.,** Neuropethia nervi optici nach Blitzschlagunfall — elektrophysiologische und computertomographische Befunde, *Klin. Monatsbl. Augenheilkd.,* 190, 56, 1987.
23. **Yost, J. W. and Holmes, F. F.,** Myoglobinuria following lightning stroke, *JAMA,* 228, 1147, 1974.

VII. PATHOPHYSIOLOGY OF THE COCHLEOVESTIBULAR SYSTEM

LaV. Bergstrom

The approximate electrical potential of a lightning bolt is 20 million V.[1]

A review of previous case reports from the 19th and 20th century literature present clinical information. Many of the victims had immediate hearing loss. Some remained completely deaf; others had partial or complete return of hearing, but the reports from the 19th and early 20th century were not precisely measured because the electric audiometer had not yet been developed. Otologists of that era, however, had complete sets of tuning forks for the various octave bands known at that time, and probably could produce a reasonable version of the audiogram.

Other patients sustained basilar skull fractures,[2] probably due to their having been thrown violently through the air to a number of feet away. Tympanic ruptures were common (Figure 1). One patient presented with the mastoid bone charred and "blown open". She developed signs of meningitis which cleared quickly with sulfanilamide, which had just come on the market.[3] Peripheral facial nerve palsy was reported in two patients.[4,5] Four children survived lightning strike, but had both cochlear and vestibular injury. The assessment was clinical; no laboratory tests were performed.[6]

An animal study using high-voltage impact resulted in tympanic membrane rupture, bleeding in the middle ear, cochlea, and cochlea aqueduct, but bleeding into the vestibular apparatus was rare.[7] The extent of injury is related to the power (watts = V × A), duration, site of entry and exit of the lightning bolt, and the position and grounding of the victim.[5-7,12] Alexander[8,9] stated that injury to vital functions varied with the path of the current, and also found that electric current passes through the body as though it were a gel.

In 1974, we reported the first known case of lightning histopathology of the ear.[10] Two possible mechanisms of lightning injury were suggested: direct effect and blast effect. The direct effect may have come through the external auditory canal. The external canal route seemed unlikely since the ossicles, especially the stapes footplate, was undisturbed, and there was no blood in the cochlea or vestibular labyrinth. A direct effect was hypothesized by injury to the central nervous system and transfer of electrical potential via the cerebrospinal fluid into the internal auditory canal, injuring the facial nerve, superior vestibular nerve, and possibly passing through the cribriform area of the fundus of the internal auditory canal into the cochlea (Figure 2). However, since the cochlear nerve, cribriform area, and modiolus were not injured, the authors concluded that cochlear injury occurred by another route or mechanism. The superior vestibular nerve showed minimal degeneration even though it lay adjacent to the facial nerve, which was very edematous. The minor pathology in the superior vestibular nerve does not explain these mild findings, and post-mortem degeneration is unlikely.

Blast effect is suggested by the fragment of cerebellum found in the internal auditory canal, the rupture of membranes in the cochlea, and the degeneration of the cochlea in our fourth patient. Blast effect at close distance would undoubtedly cause near-total deafness. Blast effect in the Vietnam war, where soldiers suffered traumatic amputations of one or more extremities, also affected the ears. All had tympanic membrane perforations which eventually were repaired. Later, the repairs broke down because a cholesteatoma was found. Seaman and Newell found implants of epithelial pearls on the promontory of the middle ear in 12% of the cases they did.[11]

The most spectacular findings in the autopsy of the temporal bone was an extreme amount of edema of the intracanalicular portion of the facial nerve which was herniated beyond "Bill's bar", an accepted surgical landmark separating the superior vestibular nerve and the facial nerve (Figure 3).

The cochlea also had extensive damage. Reissner's membrane was ruptured and collapsed onto the tectorial membrane in all cochlear turns (Figures 4 and 5). The organ of Corti was

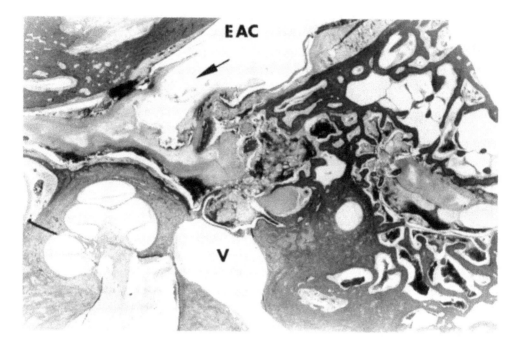

FIGURE 1. Tympanic membrane perforation (arrow) with blood and pus in middle ear and mastoid. External canal indicated by EAC and vestibule by V. (Hematoxylin-eosin, original magnification × 2.)

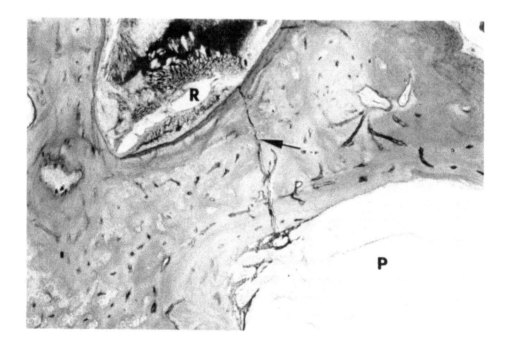

FIGURE 2. Fissure (arrow) extending from round window niche to cribriform area of ampulated end of posterior semicircular canal (P). (Hematoxylin-eosin, original magnification × 250.)

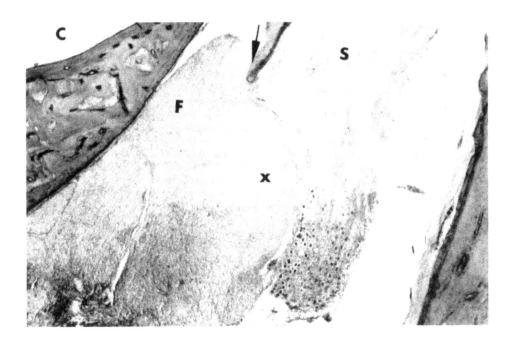

FIGURE 3. Facial nerve (F) herniated secondary to edema (X) beyond "Bill's bar" (arrow). Cochlea indicated by C and superior vestibular nerve by S. (Hematoxylin-eosin original magnification × 40.)

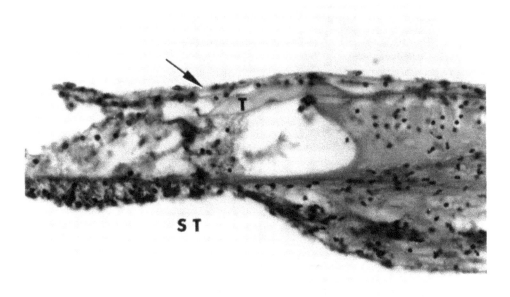

FIGURE 4. Rupture of Reissner membrane (arrow) that is doubled back on itself over tectorial membrane (T). Scala tympani indicated by ST. (Hematoxylin-eosin, original magnification × 450.)

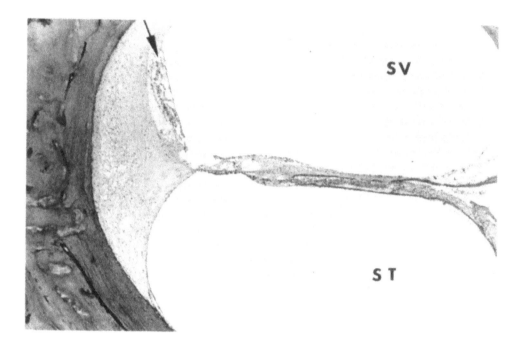

FIGURE 5. Intercellular spaces in stria vascularis (arrow) with rupture of Reissner membrane. (Hematoxylin-eosin, original magnification × 250.)

degenerated in all turns. Nerve and ganglion population were normal. The stria vascularis showed degeneration of the vas prominens and increase of intercellular spaces.

If the patients had survived, they would quite probably have had at least unilateral profound sensorineural hearing loss. The ruptured tympanic membrane, pus, blood, and keratin would likely have caused a temporary conductive hearing loss.

Most lightning stroke victims undergo autopsy, including the brain. If the institution that did the autopsy also had a temporal bone laboratory, the personnel there could remove a temporal bone, process it, and interpret the findings. This sequence of events should yield more findings than now are known.

REFERENCES

1. **Anon.,** Lightning and lightning protection, in *Encyclopedia Britannica,* Vol. 14, Chicago, 1958, 114.
2. **Thomas, J. L.,** Two cases of lightning-stroke, *Br. Med. J.,* 2, 1155, 1904.
3. **Crawford, A. S. and Hoopes, B. F.,** The surgical aspects of lightning stroke, *Surgery,* 9, 80, 1941.
4. **Bertelsen, A. S.,** Perifer facialparese efter lyntrauma, *Nord. Med.,* 6, 1602, 1958.
5. **Clark, R. O. and Brigham J. K.,** Death from lightning, *Lancet,* 2, 77, 1872.
6. **Siroky, J.,** Poraneni sluchovenko ustroji bleskem, *Cesk Otolaryngol.,* 7, 52, 1958.
7. **Loebell, H.,** The effect of electrical current upon the ear, *Arch. Ohren Usw. Heilk. Halsusw. Heilk.,* 157, 78, 1950.
8. **Alexander, L.,** Electrical injuries of the nervous system, *Arch. Neurol. Psychiatry,* 47, 179, 1941.
9. **Alexander, L.,** Electrical injuries of the nervous system, *J. Nerv. Ment. Dis.,* 94, 622, 1941.
10. **Bergstrom, L., Neblett, L. M., Sando, I., et al.,** The lightning-damaged ear, *Arch. Otolaryngol.,* 100, 117, 1974.
11. **Seaman, R. W. and Newell, R. C.,** Another etiology of middle ear cholesteatoma, *Arch. Otolaryngol.,* 94, 440, 1971.
12. **Arden, G. P. et al.,** Lightning accident at Ascot, *Br. Med. J.,* 1, 1450, 1956.

VIII. MUSCULOSKELETAL SYSTEM AND SKIN, INCLUDING BURNS

H. J. ten Duis

A. BURNS

Persons hit directly or indirectly by lightning can sustain burns ranging from transient superficial burns (commonly) to major full-thickness burns (more rarely), especially when the clothes catch fire. The seriousness of the injuries may rarely be of such an extent that they can cause hypovolemic shock and multiple organ failure.

When a subject is struck by lightning, the amount of energy that is dissipated in the tissues is dependent on the magnitude of the electric current, the body's resistance, and the current flow time. The internal body resistance (skin excluded) is relatively low because the internal tissues are more or less equivalent to an electrolyte solution. However, tissues which contain a great deal of air, such as the lungs and bowels, have a higher resistance. Based on several studies in the literature, Golde and Lee calculated a body resistance of 500 to 1000 Ω at a voltage of 1000 V and above.[1] This is in sharp contrast to the skin resistance, which varies from 10 kΩ to 1 MΩ, depending on the thickness of the skin and the degree of diaphoresis.[2,3] A thin skin which is wet by rain or perspiration will have a relatively low resistance compared with a dry, thick skin such as the palm of the hand or the sole of the foot. The resistance of the internal body tissue is small in comparison with the skin resistance, which implies that almost all the resistance to electric current is provided by the skin. Therefore, the heat production leading to burns will mainly develop at skin level, at least until skin breakdown occurs. The type of burn a lightning victim shows depends on the mechanism by which the person is affected. Six major types of burn have been identified (see Chapter 5):

1. Flash burns
2. Superficial erythema and blistering, including "flower-like" burns
3. Arborescent burns — the keraunographic marking
4. Linear burns
5. Punctate full-thickness burns, especially at entry/exit sites
6. Contact burns

Hocking and Andrews[35] have suggested, noting ten Duis et al.,[20] that the keraunographic marking and the "flower-like" burns are manifestations of the same phenomenon, and indeed may even include the linear burn. It is also noted that the flash burn is usually minor and transient. In the following discussion, the author therefore uses a classification of four major types:

1. Linear burns (4 above)
2. Keraunographic markings (2 + 3 above)
3. Contact burns (6 above)
4. Entry/exit burns (5 above)

1. Linear Burns

When a discharge (direct hit or side flash) reaches the body, the current may enter the body or spread over its surface as a surface discharge. In many cases, both pathways will be followed effectively simultaneously. The amount of current which enters the body or flows over the skin is dependent on the discharge characteristics, the breakdown strength of the skin vs. the skin surface, the presence of metal objects on the skin (e.g., zipper, necklace), and the surrounding air properties[4] (also see Chapter 3).

In the case of direct contact or side flash, a surface discharge may develop into a flashover over the body, from the site of impact to, or near to, the place where the victim makes contact with earth. If a flashover occurs, the energy dissipated within the body is greatly diminished.[4,5] This phenomenon is correlated with a high probability of survival by many authors.[1,4,6] For example, in high-voltage discharge experiments, it has been shown that when a fast flashover is observed, followed immediately by a sharp voltage and internal current drop due to the flashover, there is an increased survival rate of animals.[4] Linear burns that extend over the total length of the body are considered to be an indication that such a flashover has occurred.

In most victims of a direct hit or side flash, a burn, comprising deep-partial and full-thickness skin loss, can be observed. From the entry point of the current, in the case of a flashover, a serpiginous partial-thickness burn can often be found indicating the main tract of the current. These linear burns, which can be 1 to 10 cm wide and several decimeters long, are commonly found on the skin covering the spinal column when the victim is hit in the nape of the neck or on the anterior side of the thoracic or abdominal wall when the impact site is located at the shoulder or neck (Figure 1).[7,11] As linear burns are mostly partial-thickness burns (they show spontaneous healing in about 10 d) it is likely that they are caused by contact with the extreme heat of the electric arc rather than by heat formation in the skin as a result of skin resistance and the flow of current. It has been suggested that these burns occur along preferential paths of lower surface resistance to current flow, e.g., bands of sweat.

2. Keraunographic Markings

Keraunographic skin markings are a special kind of lightning burn, which are not real burns in a pathological respect (Figure 2). These burns are considered to be pathognomonic for lightning injuries. The shape of this erythematous lesion is often fern-like with branches scattering from a central spot, with its bright-red color contrasting with the surrounding skin.[1,12,13] The size of the individual branches is generally less than 30 cm, but may occasionally extend over a longer distance. These skin markings tend to appear shortly after the lightning impact and generally begin to fade within 12 h, and to disappear completely after 24 to 48 h without leaving any signs of residual skin changes.

The pattern of these superficial burns has been known for centuries. In 1795, Mayer, from Berlin, pointed out the similarity between their shape and those of the figures produced on Volta's electrophore.[14] (Electrical figures were described for the first time by G. R. Lichtenberg in 1777 and have since often been called Lichtenberg figures). This resemblance in manifestation was generally accepted in the 19th century, and it had been suggested that the underlying physical processes were identical.[15] Many theories have been proposed to explain the fern- or feather-like patterns. Stricker[16] and Langerhans[17] suggested that each ramified red line that could be identified near the point of lightning impact[7,16,17] could be ascribed to the injection of local branched subcutaneous blood vessels. This opinion was opposed by Rindfleisch,[18] who observed that the orientation of the skin vessels was quite different from the skin markings observed in a lightning victim[18] (Figure 3). His statement was supported by the observation that lightning marks could cross skin folds and jump from one extremity to another[14,19] (Figure 4). We now know that these skin markings will develop in a branched structure irrespective of underlying anatomical structures, such as blood vessels or nerves. They are the result of a surface discharge in which the arborization process is primarily determined by the magnitude and polarity of the discharge and secondly by skin conditions, such as perspiration and the humidity of the surrounding air.[20]

When a lightning discharge (side flash or direct strike) reaches the human body, the current may enter the body in cases where the applied voltage is not higher than the breakdown strength of the skin surface. However, when the voltage rises above this value, the current may spread over the skin as a surface discharge.

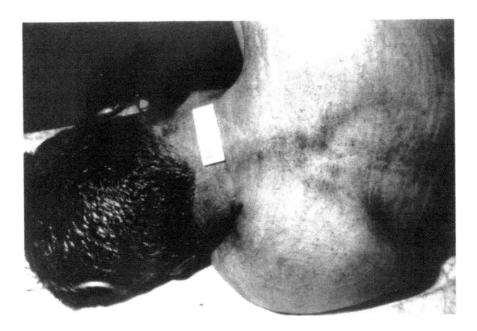

FIGURE 1. Linear burn along the spinal column. (From Unterdorfer, H. and Wykypiel, H., in *Sonderdruck Ärztliche Praxis. 4 Internationale Bergrettungsärzte Tagung*, Werk-Verlag, Munich, 1974, 63. With permission.)

A comparable situation can be created in surface discharge experiments over photographic paper.[20] When high-voltage pulses are produced over a flat earth electrode covered in photographic paper, the paper acts as an insulator and the current spreads over its surface.

Discharges of positive polarity create ramified structures identical to those observed in lightning victims, as shown in Figure 5. A very similar computer-simulated positive discharge pattern has recently been described by Niemeyer et al.[21] By combining these findings, it was concluded that the keraunographic skin markings (see Figure 2), can be related to a positive lightning surface discharge.[20] In fact, they confirm the observation made by Mayer in 1795 that "lightning can cause feather-like figures on the skin similar to those caused by positive matter on Volta's electrophore".[14]

The arborescent patterns may be modeled using "fractal" theory. A fractal is a mathematical object that manifests increasing detail with growing magnification. It implies that the magnification of a small ramification has the same general structure as a larger ramification, a property which is called self-similarity. An explanation for this fractal behavior is that in the case of a positive discharge, electrons are attracted from the surroundings in a more random manner than when a negative discharge is involved, which causes the electrons to be emitted in a more homogeneous fashion. This is illustrated in Figure 6 showing a negative discharge over photographic paper.[20] A fractal structure cannot be observed in these figures.

Interesting in this respect are the flower-like skin lesions often observed in lightning victims which also disappear within a few days[22,23] (Figure 7). That these typical figures could be related to a negative surface discharge remains rather speculative. The enigma is that a large majority of lightning-injured patients manifest arborescent patterns as opposed to flower-like patterns, yet it is known that most lightning strokes lower a negative charge to earth. It is also not uncommon for both patterns to coexist. The explanation for this enigma may lie in consideration of charge distribution during the process of a strike. Multiple current streamers may well exist in patterns of great complexity and, as far as the body is concerned, may represent both "positive" and "negative" discharges as potential equilibrates and the streamers "dance about".

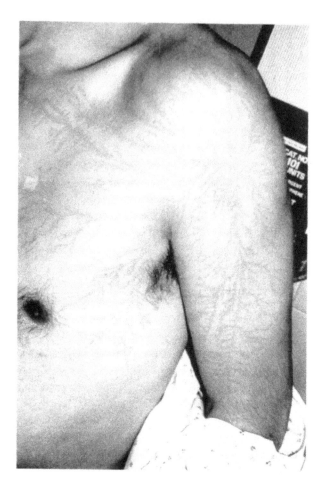

FIGURE 2. Keraunographic marking on the shoulder of a patient. (From Bartholome, C. W., Jacoby, D., and Ramchand, S. C., *Arch. Dermatol.*, 111, 1466, 1975. © American Medical Association. With permission.)

3.   Contact Burns

Contact burns may develop in areas where there is direct contact between the skin and metal objects. Metal objects worn on the skin (e.g., necklace, bracelet), incorporated into clothes (e.g., zippers), or carried in the hand are often part of the electrical circuit when a patient is struck by lightning. They may even facilitate the formation of a flashover[4] (see also Chapter 3).

The amount of heat absorbed by a metal object may be of sufficient degree that the object is melted or even evaporated. The difference in heat capacity between metals and air (metals have higher heat capacity) results in a prolonged burning time for skin in contact. The burns due to this contact are mostly of limited size; however, they are usually full thickness[24] (Figure 8).

4.   Entry- and Exit-Point Burns

The lightning return stroke has a central cross section of only a few square centimeters.[1] The temperature of the core may exceed 30,000 K for tens of microseconds.

When a victim forms part of the conducting pathway, direct contact with the heat of the electric arc as well as the formation of current heat may result in full-thickness burns at the entry point of the current. The small diameter of the central core plus the extremely short duration of the peak current flow explain why the size of the full-thickness burn is often very limited. In other cases, where contact with the electric arc is included in a splash, a relatively large surface burn

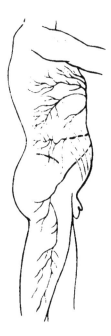

FIGURE 3. Lichtenberg figures described by Rindfleisch. Note the different orientation from epigastric and axillary (skin) vessels.

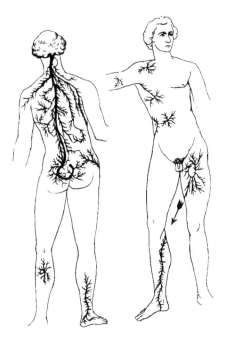

FIGURE 4. Keraunographic markings described by Mayer in 1795.

of 10- to 20-cm diameter results. The burn is usually one of deep partial thickness, sometimes with blistering, sometimes with typical brown coloring of the skin.[9,16,24] In the case of a flashover, a linear burn may radiate away from the contact point of the current.

There is a great deal of resemblance between splash burns from lightning and those associated with high-voltage electrical accidents when an electric arc develops between the victim and an

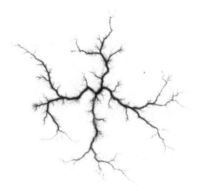

FIGURE 5. Positive discharge recorded on photographic paper. (From ten Duis, H. J., Klasen, H. J., Nijsten, M. W. N., and Pietronero, L., *Burns*, 13, 141, 1987. With permission.)

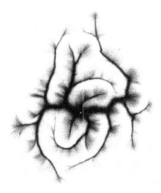

FIGURE 6. Negative discharge recorded on photographic paper. (From ten Duis, H. J., Klasen, H. J., Nijsten, M. W. N., and Pietronero, L., *Burns*, 13, 141, 1987. With permission.)

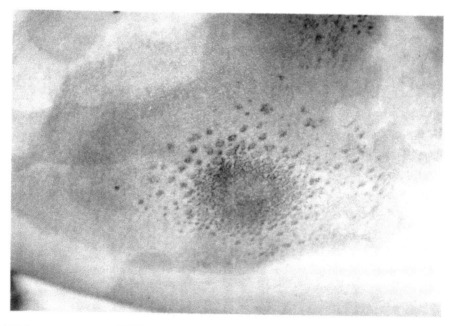

FIGURE 7. Superficial flower-like burn on a 10-year-old boy. (From McCrady-Kahn, V. L. and Kahn, A. M., *West. J. Med.*, 134, 215, 1981. Reprinted by permission of the Western Journal of Medicine.)

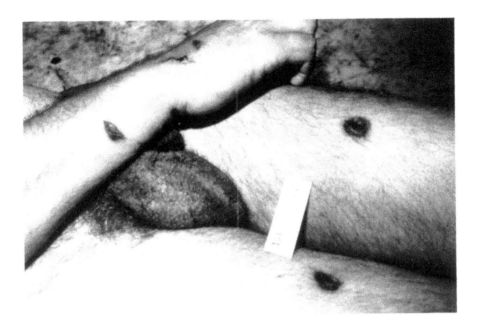

FIGURE 8. Contact burns on upper legs and forearm. (From Unterdorfer, H. and Wykypiel, H., in *Sonderdruck Ärztliche Praxis. 4 Internationale Bergrettungsärzte Tagung*. Werk-Verlag, Munich, 1974, 63. With permission.)

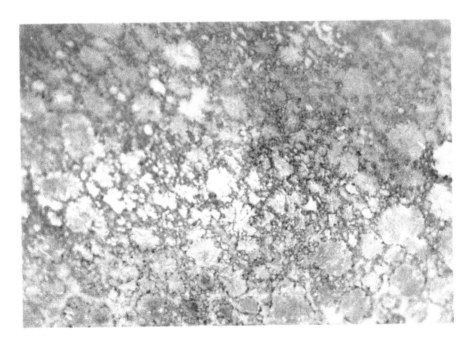

FIGURE 9. Splash burn on a lightning victim. (From McCrady-Kahn, V. L. and Kahn, A. M., *West. J. Med.*, 134, 215, 1981. Reprinted by permission of the Western Journal of Medicine.)

electric wire. The duration of the electric discharge is usually much longer than in a lightning discharge and consequently results in a relatively larger and deeper burned surface area.

The clinical picture of a splash burn is characterized by an almost completely evaporated horny layer of the epidermis (Figures 9 and 10). Shortly after the lightning impact, these burns

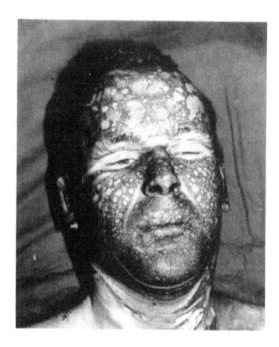

FIGURE 10. Splash burn by high-voltage electric arc.

can be diagnosed as being partial thickness. However, reevaluation after 24 to 48 h will reveal that they have become full-thickness burns. This is the result of an impaired circulation of the deep dermal layer due to edema formation. Recirculation normally takes place within 1 week and is illustrated by spontaneous reepithelialization within 2 to 3 weeks. It is important to be aware of this pathophysiological process, because misinterpretation might influence the making of surgical therapeutic decisions.

The skin lesions at the exit points of the current are mostly small full-thickness burns and result from the concentration of current. They can be found near or at places where the victim makes contact with the earth potential, such as the sole of the foot, the ankle, or the lower leg.[9,24,25]

Full-thickness burns over a large surface area are usually the result of the ignition of clothing secondary to a direct hit, side flash, or flashover. These burns might be of such an extent that they can cause hypovolemic shock and secondary death, as is also the case with genuine burns.

B. MUSCULOSKELETAL INJURIES

Musculoskeletal injuries due to lightning impact originate via two, principally different injury mechanisms:

1.   Mechanical injuries
2.   Current flow-related injuries

1. Mechanical Injuries

The sudden onset of a very high current flowing through the body may cause maximal muscle contraction. This may result in ruptures of skeletal muscles as well as fractures of long bones. Moreover, the victim is often thrown for meters. When this is the case and the person falls down or hits a solid object, secondary musculoskeletal injuries may occur. A review of the lightning literature has shown that this is a rare cause of soft tissue and skeletal injuries.[9]

2. Current Flow-Related Injuries

Current flow injuries are a common observation in high-tension electrical injuries: a high current flowing for a considerable time (seconds) induces heat coagulation and coagulation necrosis of soft tissues.[2,26] The amount of heat generation is dependent on the voltage applied, current flow (amperage), internal body resistance, and flow time. Because a direct correlation also exists with the diameter of the object through which the current is flowing, serious damage is often sustained to muscles and tendons of the forearms and hands as well as to the lower legs and feet. Thus, in high-tension injuries, it is not unusual for compartment syndromes to develop which require extensive decompression fasciotomies.[26]

In contrast, in lightning accidents, the initial current which flows through the body is usually much higher than that involved in high-voltage electrical accidents. The extremely short duration of most lightning current impulses limits the energy dissipation in the body and consequently the heat generation in the tissues, except in a highly localized channel. This might be the reason why compartment syndromes and muscle injuries related to current flow have seldom been mentioned in the lightning literature.[27-29]

The pathophysiological aspects of soft tissue necrosis caused by an electrical injury are comparable to those observed in crush injuries. Soft tissue injuries involving a great deal of damage to the muscle cells, e.g., rhabdomyolysis, have serious consequences for the patient. During the process of rhabdomyolysis, several kinds of breakdown products are released into the circulation. The most important proteins are myoglobin, creatinine phosphokinase (CPK), aldolase, aspartate aminotransferase (ASAT), alanine aminotransferase (ALAT), and lactate dehydrogenase (LDH).

The clinical picture of rhabdomyolysis, i.e., acute renal failure and shock, is strongly related to high levels of myoglobin in the circulating blood as well as to the occurrence of myoglobinuria. The potential nephrotoxicity of myoglobin and its derivatives has been studied extensively. It is generally accepted that free circulating heme pigments, such as myoglobin and hemoglobin, are nontoxic in themselves. However, they may induce nephropathy in two different ways:

1. Tubular obstruction and subsequent tubular necrosis by the precipitation of high molecular heme proteins
2. A direct nephrotoxicity effect of myoglobin in the case of systemic acidosis or decreased renal blood flow[30]

Therefore, urine alkalization and volume-forced diuresis is widely recommended in treatment protocols for high-voltage injuries.

It is worthwhile noting that hemolysis of 10 to 30% of the circulating blood volume is observed in patients with severe muscle injuries as well as in patients with major full-thickness burns.[31] This is the reason why in the dark-colored urine, myoglobin and hemoglobin can often be determined.

The breakdown of muscle tissue will also result in the release of lysosomal enzymes, bioamines, and cell stroma products, as well as phosphate and uric acid. Especially when there has been a long, warm ischemic period, large amounts of lactate and potassium may be set free.

The release of large quantities of cell disintegration products and metabolites will give rise to the induction of an acute phase reaction. Macrophages and endothelial cells induce fever via the production of interleukines. Complement activation, PMN (polymorphonuclear leukocyte) and platelet aggregation, PMN-elastase release, and free oxygen-radical formation result in capillary endothelial damage. Consequently, the leakage of intravascular fluids leads to the formation of edema and, if not treated adequately, to shock.

In victims of lightning injury who are found to be suffering from myoglobinuria, it remains questionable whether severe limb ischemia also contributes to the muscle damage. Transient limb ischemia, due to arterial spasm or vasomotor nerve distrubances, is theoretically possible.[32-34] Recirculation of the limb may lead to progressive muscle swelling and may rarely require adequate surgical treatment (fasciotomy).[11,29] Only then can local as well as systemic circulatory impairment be sufficiently prevented.

Myoglobin-related nephropathy and the full-blown picture of acute pathophysiological disturbances have only been described in a few reports on lightning injuries.[8,9,27] As mentioned above, the incidence is probably much lower than in high-voltage electrical injuries due to the smaller amount of energy dissipated in the tissues.

REFERENCES

1. **Golde, R. H. and Lee, W. R.**, Death by lightning, *Inst. Electr. Eng. Rev.*, 123, 1163, 1976.
2. **Jellinek, S.**, *Der Elektrische Unfall*, Franz Deuticke, Leipzig, 1927, 75.
3. **Schaefer, H.**, Allgemeine physiologische Theorie des elektrischen Herztodes, in *Der Elektrunfall*, Brinkmann, K. and Schaefer, H., Eds., Springer Verlag, New York, 1982, 181.
4. **Ohashi, M., Kitagawa, N., and Ishikawa, T.**, Lightning injury caused by discharges accompanying flashovers — a clinical and experimental study of death and survival, *Burns*, 12, 496, 1986.
5. **Kitagawa, N., Kinoshita, K., and Ishikawa, T.**, Discharge experiments using dummies and rabbits simulating lightning strokes on human bodies, *Int. J. Biometeorol.*, 17, 239, 1972.
6. **Cooper, M. A.**, Prognostic signs for death, *Ann. Emerg. Med.*, 9, 134, 1980.
7. **Stricker, W.**, Neue Untersuchungen und Beobachtungen über die Wirkung des Blitzes auf den menschlichen Körper, in *Archiv. für pathologische Anatomie und Physiologie und für klinische Medicin*, Bd. XXVIII, Virchow, R., Ed., Georg Reimer Verlag, Berlin, 1863, 552.
8. **Hellbach**, Beobachtung einer Verletzung durch den Blitz, *Corresp. Bl. Vereins Nassau'scher Aerzte*, 9, 77, 1859.
9. **Krauland, W.**, Schäden und Todesfälle durch Blitzschlag, *Dtsche. Z. Gerichtl. Med.*, 40, 298, 1951.
10. **Strasser, E. J., Davis, R. M., and Menchey, M. J.**, Lightning injuries, *J. Trauma*, 17, 315, 1977.
11. **Amy, B. W., McManus, W. F., Goodwin, C. W., and Pruitt, B. A.**, Lightning injury with survival in five patients, *JAMA*, 253, 243, 1985.
12. **Bartholome, C. W., Jacoby, D., and Ramchand, S. C.**, Cutaneous manifestations of lightning injury, *Arch. Dermatol.*, 111, 1466, 1975.
13. **Keller**, Fälle von Blitzverletzung, *Dtsche. Med. Wochenschr.*, 39, 1233, 1917.
14. **Mayer, R.**, *Neuen Bemerkungen und Erfahrungen zur Wundarzneikunst und Arzneigelehrtheit*, Berlin III Theil, 1795.
15. **Pfaffe, M.**, Blitz, in *Gehlers Physikalisches Woerterbuch, neue Bearbeitung*, Leipzig, 1825, 1016.
16. **Stricker, W.**, Die Wirkung des Blitzes auf den Menschlichen Körper, in *Archiv für pathologische Anatomie und Physiologie und für klinische Medicin*, Bd. XX, Virchow, R., Ed., Georg Reimer Verlag, Berlin, 1860, 45.
17. **Langerhans, T.**, *Archiv für pathologische Anatomie und Physiologie und für klinische Medicin*, Bd. XXIV, Virchow, R., Ed., Georg Reimer Verlag, Berlin, 1862, 200.
18. **Rindfleisch, E.**, Ein Fall von Blitzschlag, in *Archiv für pathologische Anatomie und Physiologie und für klinische Medicin*, Bd. XXV, Virchow, R., Ed., Georg Reimer Verlag, Berlin, 1862, 417.
19. **Sonnenburg, E. and Tschmarke, P.**, Verbrennung und Allgemeinschädigung durch elektrische Energie, in *Neue Deutsche Chirurgie*, Bd. 17, Von Burns, P., Ed., Ferdinand Enke Verlag, Stuttgart, 1915, 74.
20. **ten Duis, H. J., Klasen, H. J., Nijsten, M. W. N., and Pietronero, L.**, Superficial lightning injuries — their fractal shape and origin, *Burns*, 13, 141, 1987.
21. **Niemeyer, L., Pietronero, L., and Wiesmann, H. J.**, Fractal dimension of dielectric breakdown, *Phys. Rev. Lett.*, 52, 1033, 1984.
22. **McCrady-Kahn, V. L. and Kahn, A. M.**, Lightning burns, *West. J. Med.*, 134, 215, 1981.
23. **Edland, J. F.**, Electrical injuries and lightning, in *Forensic Pathology*, Castle House, Kent, 1980, 111.
24. **Unterdorfer, H. and Wykypiel, H.**, Statistik und Morphologie tödlicher Blitzunfälle, in *Sonderdruck Ärztliche Praxis, 4 Internationale Bergrettungsärzte Tagung*, Werk-Verlag, Munich, 1974, 63.
25. **Milward, T. M.**, Prolonged gastric dilatation as a complication of lightning injury, *Burns*, 1, 175, 1974.
26. **Mann, R. J. and Wallquist, J. M.**, Early decompression fasciotomy in the treatment of high-voltage electrical burns of the extremities, *South. Med. J.*, 68, 1103, 1975.
27. **Yost, J. W. and Holmes, F. F.**, Myoglobinuria following lightning stroke, *JAMA*, 228, 1147, 1974.
28. **Apfelberg, D. B., Masters, F. W., and Robinson, D. W.**, Pathophysiology and treatment of lightning injuries, *J. Trauma*, 14, 453, 1974.
29. **Spielberger, M. and Flora, G.**, Blitzunfall: Sofortmassnahmen und klinische Behandlung, in *Sonderdruck Ärztliche Praxis, 4 Internationale Bergrettungsärzte Tagung*, 1974, 78.
30. **Knochel, J. P.**, Rhabdomyolysis and myoglobinuria, *Sem. Nephr.*, 1, 75, 1981.

31. **Dijkema, H. E. and Klasen, H. J.,** Bloedtransfusie in de acute fase van brandwonden?, *Ned Militair Geneeskd Tijdschr.* 41, 64, 1988.
32. **Lynch, M. J. G. and Shorthouse, P. H.,** Injuries and death from lightning, *Lancet,* 1, 473, 1949.
33. **Currens, J. H.,** Arterial spasm and transient paralysis resulting from lightning striking on airplane, *J. Aviat. Med.,* 16, 275, 1945.
34. **ten Duis, H. J., Klasen, H. J., and Reenalda, P. E.,** Keraunoparalysis, a "specific" lightning injury, *Burns,* 12, 54, 1985.
35. **Hocking, B. and Andrews, C. J.,** Fractals and lightning injury, *Med. J. Austr.,* 150 (7), 409, 1989.

IX. RENAL, METABOLIC, HEMATOLOGIC, AND GASTROINTESTINAL SYSTEMS

C. J. Andrews

A. METABOLIC CONSEQUENCES

One of the major enigmas of lightning injury is the widely claimed phenomenon of documented survival with minimal deficit after prolonged unresuscitated cardiac arrest. This contention appears untenable and flies in the face of accepted findings, where it is agreed that cerebral anoxia leads to permanent damage after 4 min of lost perfusion.

To explain this, it has been proposed that after a strike all metabolism ceases, and that the lack of metabolic demand means that lack of perfusion is immaterial. This proposition receives most currency due to its espousal by Taussig.[1] Since then, it has often been repeated (e.g., References 4, 5, 19, and 20). Although the notion is widely attributed to Taussig, in fact, it predates her widely quoted paper, although not in such definite form. Former reports include those of Critchley,[21] Jellinek,[2] and Ravitch et al.[8]

Jex-Blake[22] provides a fascinating account of the history of views on lightning injury which include views on resuscitation. Many are obviously speculative, but an equivalent of cessation of metabolism does not seem to have been mentioned at that time. The first time that the proposal was made is attributed by Critchley[21] to Jellinek.[23,24] The effect is described in this initial work as "suspended animation". The notion that respiration and circulation were intimately involved with survival had long been current (see Jex-Blake), and the necessity to reestablish both was known. Critchley[21] was the first to suggest that resuscitation after "several hours" of demonstrated cessation of respiration and circulation was possible, based not on personal experience, but on other reports. The reason for the resuscitability was said to be that the victim was in "suspended animation". Lynch and Shorthouse[3] provide a similar reference to Jellinek and Critchley, and are perhaps the first to question the phenomenon, saying that a certain German expert, Alvensleben, was skeptical about resuscitation after more than one half hour of suspended animation. Nonetheless, they recognized that reports of long-term suspended animation being reversed do exist, but more often after technical electrical injury than lightning injury.

Ravitch et al.,[8] also summarized earlier by Morikawa and Steichen,[9] provide a report of such a case. A child was struck and immediately after the strike was questionably thought to demonstrate a pulse, but no respiratory effort. He was given manual respiration for about 10 min, and this was then ceased, although a pulse was still thought to be present. Seven minutes later, he arrived at a hospital by ambulance with no successful pulmonary inflation for all that time and was found to be pulseless. An open thoracotomy indicated an asystolic heart with no bleeding from the wound. After an additional 3 min — 20 min after the strike — cardiac action was restored and, ultimately, successful restoration of function was achieved.

This sequence of events was later cited by Taussig[1] as her only support for the hypothesis of immediate "cessation of metabolism" in lightning strike, thus allowing prolonged arrest with successful later resuscitation. The example is therefore not a good one in this connection. It would seem more to fit the sequence of events described by Andrews et al.,[25] in which experimental data supported the hypothesis of primary cardiac arrest and respiratory arrest, followed by cardiac recovery and secondary hypoxic arrest.

Based only on the case above, Taussig strongly asserts that all body metabolism ceases after a lightning strike. The assertion has then been repeated by several authors in a form giving it status as accepted theory. There is no experimental evidence to support the contention of cessation of metabolism, and it is seriously questioned by those with any experience in treating such patients (see References 27 to 29).

Several reports commonly regarded as supporting the notion of such recovery (see, e.g., Kleiner and Wilkin,[5] who state that at least six published cases support the contention) bear further examination, e.g., Kravitz et al.,[10] Kleinot et al.,[29] Yost and Holmes,[12] Burda,[30] and Hanson and McIlwraith.[11] In each of these cases, there was certainly a prolonged period of cardiac arrest, but early resuscitation was also attempted to a greater or lesser degree within the knowledge of the day. Most often, this was respiratory support only. In the given reports, there was no documented period of prolonged hypoperfusion that would require the induction of a hypothesis to suggest low metabolic demand. The fact that recovery was achieved, at least temporarily, indicates more the success of the resuscitation attempted. It may be that such resuscitation was ineffective, given more recent knowledge of the techniques of emergency first aid, and if so, one must look further for explanation of the documented survival, but the reports concerned are not couched in this light. That another explanation is required is only necessary if it is presumed that ineffective attempted resuscitation occurred, and certainly not as a result of documented prolonged unresuscitated arrest. There is no evidence to support recovery from lightning injury after the accepted period of a few minutes of unresuscitated arrest has passed, and it is on this misconception that many of the claims for a state of metabolic standstill have been made.

Indeed, Andrews et al.[28] have stated that the cessation of metabolism hypothesis, though implausible, has not been supplanted by anything better — if, indeed, one accepts that the phenomenon occurs at all. Although the evidence is at best questionable, as above, for recovery after a documented prolonged unresuscitated arrest, the dogma is still widely held. At best, survival after prolonged unconsciousness with attempted resuscitation is supported by the literature. It is the aim of the following discussion to propose a more plausible alternative than the currently held version of cessation of metabolism on the assumption that resuscitation was less than effective — given that it was generally noncardiac and involved techniques of respiratory support that have been supplanted.

1.   An Alternative Hypothesis to Cessation of Metabolism

Andrews et al.[31] have proposed an alternative to the cessation of metabolism hypothesis. They note prolongation of the QT interval in lightning injury, as do Palmer[17] and Divakov.[18] They also note that this prolongation is a general phenomenon in lightning injury. QT prolongation is known to predispose to Torsade de Pointe ventricular tachycardia (VT). Further, they give evidence of hyperadrenergic effects on the myocardium in the form of patchy myocardial necrosis, pulmonary edema. The lightning-injured state is known to be hyperadrenergic.

A speculative hypothesis of subsequent cardiac behavior after the primary asystolic arrest was outlined, especially where some form of respiratory support had been given. It was first note that QT prolongation highly predisposes to Torsade de Pointe VT and that QT prolongation is a strong feature of lightning injury. In that state, pulses will be absent. A victim will therefore *appear* to be in cardiac arrest. Nonetheless, it is known that cardiac output may still be just present in this or, indeed, other forms of VT, although not, of course, anywhere near full function.

Subsequent events, it was postulated, depend on catecholamine levels in the individual case. Given that a hyperadrenergic state exists, Torsade VT may well terminate in cardiac recovery, at least initially. Sufficient catecholamine may arrive at the heart to stimulate recovery, and a good rhythm and output may occur and be maintained. If sufficient catecholamine levels persist, the heart may proceed to secondary hypoxic arrest, as outlined above. It is conceivable that if catecholamine levels fall subsequent to this degree of recovery, further episodes of Torsade VT may then occur and the process may cycle.

Alternatively, if catecholamine levels are not high, the heart may again lapse into bradycardia and/or episodic Torsade VT, since QT prolongation will still exist. Episodes of Torsade VT and bradycardia may be sufficient to maintain perfusion just sufficient to maintain viability.

In either case, and the balance may depend on catecholamine levels in individual cases, a period relatively longer than the classically allowed few minutes in cardiac arrest will appear to have occurred. The victim may appear pulseless and lifeless, as if cardiac arrest due to ventricular fibrillation has occurred. If ventilation without cardiac support occurs, as has been reported in the literature especially in the days prior to external cardiac compression, then the state may persist for some time, giving an illusion of recovery after prolonged arrest.

Thus, an alternative hypothesis to cessation of metabolism has been proposed, its operation depending on catecholamine levels, and enhanced by varying degrees of artificial ventilation.

2. Other Metabolic Effects

The hypertension and tachycardia seen in lightning injury, and sometimes peripheral vasoconstriction, are postulated to be due to sympathetic overactivity.[10,11] Kravitz et al.[10] state that this is due to direct adrenal stimulation, whereas others say its genesis is central. There has been only one set of documented catecholamine assays to verify this state.[11] The assays were elevated by an unstated amount. The dominant catecholamine was adrenaline.

B. GASTROINTESTINAL SYSTEM

Gastric dilatation and bowel bruising and perforation have been reported.[11] The genesis of perforation has been ascribed to superexpansion of intestinal gas, although reported perforations have been multiple and small. Severe bruising has been ascribed to blast contusion, and dilatation to functional ileus formation. Gastrointestinal bleeding may be similarly based, although stress ulceration is a common phenomenon in many forms of trauma, especially cerebral trauma.

C. RENAL PATHOPHYSIOLOGY

Most reports describe at least transient myoglobinuria (e.g., References 12 and 13), although never of the significance that exists with major traumatic and electrical muscle damage. In the latter cases, the myoglobin results from extensive heat and crush-damaged muscle releasing myoglobin pigment into the circulation. Yost[12] reports it to be surprisingly rare in lightning injury, and notes that it may result from vascular emboli, vigorous muscle contraction, cardiac injury, systemic hypoxia, and resuscitation effort.

Regardless of its etiology, myoglobinuria carries the threat of acute renal failure. There is debate on whether this acute failure results from interference with tubular ion transport, myoglobin cytotoxicity (although this is questioned[14]), or myoglobin casts blocking ducts and eroding tubules. Two consequences of myoglobinuria are thought to be that (1) free hemoglobin increases glomerular permeability to myoglobin, which, in turn, causes constriction of renal arterioles, depriving the cortex of blood, and (2) tubule occlusion with casts causes pressure ischemia in the cortex. ten Duis (q.v.) discusses this matter further.

Anderson et al.[14] state that while myoglobin itself is not nephrotoxic, other muscle breakdown products are, and in a setting of hypovolemia which often accompanies muscle injury, renal pressure ischemia (as above) may heighten this toxicity.

D. HEMATOLOGICAL SYSTEM

Hematological signs have been outlined in Chapter 4. The case of Erythemia di Guglielmo and AML is an isolated report and only temporally related to a lightning strike. Eng[15] states that "although it was not proved that the lightning injury caused or precipitated the blood changes, it is thought not to be improbable". No pathogenetic mechanism is advanced. As AML is a known transition from Erythemia di Guglielmo, it would seem that the genesis of the latter from the lightning stroke is the phenomenon that still needs explanation.

DIC has been reported,[16] with its genesis being in a standard setting of prolonged shock, burns, and myocardial necrosis.

REFERENCES

1. **Taussig, H.,** 'Death' from lightning and the possibility of living again, *Ann. Int. Med.,* 68, 1345, 1968.
2. **Jellinek, S.,** Death by lightning (lett.), *Br. Med. J.,* December, 714, 1942.
3. **Lynch, M. and Shorthouse, P. H.,** Injuries and death from lightning, *Lancet,* 1, 473, 1949.
4. **Bartholome, C. W., Jacoby, D., and Ramchand, S.,** Cutaneous manifestations of lightning injury, *Arch. Dermatol.,* 111, 1466, 1975.
5. **Kleiner, J. P. and Wilkin, J. H.,** Cardiac effects of lightning stroke, *JAMA,* 240, 2757, 1978.
6. **Apfelberg, D. B., Masters, F. W., and Robinson, D. W.,** Pathophysiology of treatment of lightning injuries, *J. Trauma,* 14(6), 453, 1974.
7. **Moran, K. T., Thupari, J. N., and Munster, A. M.,** Electric and lightning induced cardiac arrest reversed by cardiopulmonary resuscitation (lett.), *JAMA,* 255(16), 2157, 1986b.
8. **Ravitch, M. M., Lane, R., Safar, P., Steichen, F., and Knowles, P.,** Lightning stroke, *N. Engl. J. Med.,* 264(1), 36, 1961.
9. **Morikawa, S. and Steichen, F.,** Successful resuscitation after 'death' from lightning, *Anesthesiology,* 21(2), 222, 1960.
10. **Kravitz, H., Wasserman, M. J., Valaitis, J., et al.,** Lightning injury, *Am. J. Dis. Child.,* 131, 413, 1977.
11. **Hansen, G. C. and McIlwraith, G. R.,** Lightning injury: two case histories and a review of management, *Br. Med. J.,* 4, 271, 1973.
12. **Yost, J. W. and Holmes, F. F.,** Myoglobinuria following lightning stroke, *JAMA,* 228, 1147, 1974.
13. **Smith, J.,** Lightning Injuries, *J. Emerg. Nurs.,* 9(5), 248, 1983.
14. **Anderson, R. J. and Schrier, R. W.,** Acute failure, in *Harrison's Principles of Internal Medicine,* 11th ed., Braunwald, E. et al., Eds., McGraw-Hill, New York, 1987.
15. **Eng, L. and Sinnadurai, C.,** Syndrome of Erythemia di Guglielmo after lightning injury with autoimmune antibodies and terminating in acute monocytic leukaemia, *Blood,* 25(5), 845, 1965.
16. **Ekoe, J. M., Cunningham, M., Jaques, O., et al.,** Disseminated intravascular coagulation and acute myocardial necrosis caused by lightning, *Int. Care Med.,* 11, 160, 1985.
17. **Palmer, A. B. D.,** Lightning injury causing prolongation of the Q-T interval, *Post. Med. J.,* 63, 891, 1987.
18. **Divakov, G. M.,** ECG changes in persons struck by lightning, *Klin. Meditsima (Mosc.),* 95, 1966 (trans. from Russian).
19. **Nesmith, M. A.,** A case of lightning stroke, *J. Fla. Med. Assoc.,* 58, 36, 1971, quoted in Hanson et al. (1973).
20. **Msonge, B. and Evans, R., L.,** Lightning stroke on Ukerewe Island, *East Afr. Med. J.,* 53(6), 350, 1976.
21. **Critchley, M.,** Neurological effects of lightning and of electricity, *Lancet,* 1, 68, 1934.
22. **Jex-Blake, A. J.,** Goulstonian Lectures: Death by electric currents and by lightning, *Br. Med. J.,* 425–430, 492–498, 548–552, 601–603, Mar. 1, 8, 15, 22, 1913.
23. **Jellinek, S.,** *Wien Klin. Wschr.,* 45, 37, 1932a; quoted in Lynch et al., op. cit.
24. **Jellinek, S.,** *Electrische Verletzungen,* Leipzig, 1932b; quoted in Lynch et al., op. cit.
25. **Andrews, C. J. and Darveniza, M.,** Effects of lightning on mammalian tissue, *Proc. 3rd Int. Conf. Lightning Stat. Elec.,* Bath, Sept. 1989, ERA Technology, Leatherhead, Surrey.
26. **Cooper, M. A.,** personal communication.
27. **ten Duis, H. J.,** personal communication.
28. **Andrews, C. J., Darveniza, M., and Mackerras, D.,** Lightning injury: a review of clinical aspects, pathophysiology, and treatment, *Adv. Trauma,* 4, 241, 1989.
29. **Kleinot, S., Klachki, D. M., and Keeley, K. J.,** The cardiac effects of Lightning injury, *S. Afr. Med. J.,* 40, 1141, 1966.
30. **Burda, C. A.,** Electrocardiographic changes in lightning stroke, *Am. Heart J.,* 72, 521, 1966.
31. **Andrews, C. J. and Colquhoun, D. M.,** The QT interval in lightning strike and its implications for the "cessation of metabolism" hypothesis, *J. Wild. Med.,* submitted.

Chapter 7

TREATMENT OF LIGHTNING INJURY

TABLE OF CONTENTS

I. INTRODUCTION AND FIRST AID

Mary Ann Cooper

A. INITIAL OVERVIEW

Lightning injuries generally can be grouped into three classes of severity: mild, moderate, and severe. The prognosis and treatment depend on the severity of injury and the presenting signs that the patient exhibits.

1. Mild Injury

The mildly injured patient is often just stunned by the stroke. They usually are awake and able to respond to questions, although they may be confused and amnesic for the event, and continue to have difficulty with short-term memory assimilation for a few hours or days after the incident. They may complain of temporary deafness or blindness, but seldom demonstrate cutaneous burns or paralysis. They will often have rupture of at least one eardrum. Vital signs are usually stable, although an occasional patient may exhibit transient mild hypertension that usually does not require treatment. Recovery is usually gradual, but they may complain of paresthesia and muscular pain that may last for several weeks or months.

2. Moderate Injury

The moderately injured patient may be disoriented, combative, or comatose. They often have keraunoparalysis, with paralysis of the lower and sometimes upper extremities that lasts for several hours. The extremities that are affected will appear blue, mottled, pale, and pulseless, and it is difficult to differentiate this from true hypovolemic shock unless the blood pressure is evaluated by Doppler. If true hypotension exists, the patient should be evaluated for spinal injuries and other sources of shock such as blunt abdominal injuries or massive fractures. First- and second-degree burns may be present, but more commonly develop over the next several hours after injury. Tympanic membrane injury is common. These victims may have suffered a temporary cardiopulmonary standstill with the stroke and recovered spontaneously, and should be evaluated with an electrocardiogram. Rarely, seizures may occur in these victims. These patients are highly likely to survive. However, they may also have permanent sequelae such as sleep disorders, paresthesias, generalized weakness, personality changes, and difficulty with fine motor functions and some mental functions.

3. Severe Injury

Severely injured victims often present in cardiac arrest with either ventricular standstill or fibrillation. Cardiac resuscitation may, on occasion, be successful. While the lightning literature is rampant with the single case report of survival after a prolonged resuscitation, there is no reason to believe that this is the norm and that prolonged resuscitative measures will benefit those who do not respond to routine advanced cardiac life-support measures. Direct brain damage may occur from the stroke or as a result of hypoxia secondary to the cardiac arrest. Blunt trauma, skull fracture, and intracranial injuries are more common in these patients. The prognosis for recovery in this group is usually poor except for those who rapidly respond to resuscitative measures.

B. FIRST AID

The victim of lightning stroke may suffer a range of injuries (see Chapter 5), from being temporarily stunned to full cardiac arrest. There may be multiple victims in any incident. The emergency treatment in the field, then, must be varied and appropriate to the level of injury as well as to the number of victims. This section will discuss the immediate things that a bystander can do, the approach to a multiple casualty situation, and the actions that emergency medical personnel (paramedics and emergency medical technicians) should take when they arrive at the scene.

1.   Bystander Response — Evaluating the Victim

The victim of lightning stroke who is breathing and talking has an excellent prognosis and usually needs only to be evaluated at the hospital to rule out cardiac, neurologic, burn, otologic, or ophthalmic damage. The role of the bystander who witnesses or happens onto the scene of a lightning incident should be to assess the situation and, in the minimally injured victim, primarily to provide supportive psychological and physical care for the patient, urging them to be transported to the hospital for evaluation and orienting them to what has happened, since the victim may have anterograde as well as some retrograde amnesia, may be quite confused, and is often unable to assimilate new information for a few hours or days or make logical decisions about their well-being.

The victim who is found unconscious must be assessed for the presence of pulse and respiration. It is extremely rare for a person with pulse and respiration to die, although they may still have significant injuries and sequelae. The pulse should be sought centrally in the carotid or femoral area, since the more severely injured victim may have intense vascular spasm of his extremities which makes the pulse very difficult to find. If the victim is not breathing and does not have a pulse, cardiopulmonary resuscitation should be started immediately.

The current theory connecting lightning and cardiac injury is that lightning acts as cosmic countershock, sending the heart into ventricular standstill (asystole), and that the heart will often resume its rhythm due to the heart's property of automaticity, but that the accompanying respiratory arrest is more long lasting, leading to a secondary cardiac arrest and arrhythmias due to hypoxia. This theory has come about from anecdotal literature and has not been confirmed by experimental data, although Andrews and Darveniza (Proc. Int. Conf. Lightning Stat. Elec., ERA Technology, Surrey, U.K., 1989) have recently provided qualified support for this process in an animal model. If the theory is true, the victim has the best chance of recovery if they receive immediate ventilation and/or chest compressions, as indicated by the victim's vital signs.

As the rescuer is starting cardiopulmonary resuscitation, he should ensure that someone else is summoning a medical response team. Unfortunately, if the victim is in a wilderness area where timely rescue is unlikely, prolonged basic cardiopulmonary resuscitation is not only impractical, but also may not be effective in either resuscitating the victim or in preventing hypoxic brain damage.

For the nonarrested victim, the airway, if obstructed, should be opened with the chin lift or jaw thrust maneuver, not with extension of the neck since spinal injuries have been reported to occur with lightning injuries. If there is any suspicion that the victim has fallen or been thrown a distance in connection with the lightning stroke, the victim should be left where they are until spinal precautions (backboard and cervical immobilization) can be done in order to protect the victim from further harm due to movement of potentially unstable fractures. The only exception to this would be if the victim is in immediate danger of suffering life-threatening harm for some reason, such as having a seizure near the edge of a precipice.

Blunt injuries, spinal cord trauma, and closed head injuries have been reported, and the patient should be evaluated for them. Any fractures or dislocations should be splinted. Burns, if there are any, may be covered by a dry, clean cloth or dressing pending arrival of prehospital care personnel. Hemorrhage, a rare event with lightning injury, should be controlled with direct pressure over the wound, not by tourniquets or other methods of vascular compression.

A victim who is having a seizure should be protected from injuring themselves. Since most seizures resolve on their own in less that 1 min, trying to insert something into the victim's mouth is not only unnecessary, but may be dangerous to both the victim and the rescuer.

2. Response to Multiple Victims

If the rescuer is presented with several victims, he must make a decision as to where he will expend his efforts and must *triage* the victims. As stated earlier, the victims who are breathing and have a pulse, regardless of the state of consciousness, are generally going to do well. The victims without pulse and respiration are the ones on whom the rescuer can have the most impact. While victims with lesser injuries will need to be tended to eventually, the rescuer's immediate efforts should be applied to those who are most critically ill. Other, nonskilled bystanders may be employed to monitor the less critically ill victims.

3. Prehospital Care Response

When emergency medical services (EMS) personnel arrive on the scene, they should assess the scene for continuing danger to the victims, other rescuers, and themselves, and secure the area accordingly. They will need to determine the number of victims, triage them for care, determine the care that has already been rendered, plan their response according to their findings, and call for additional help, if necessary.

For the single conscious victim, the guidelines as noted above apply. Simple reassurance and transport for medical evaluation are all that are usually necessary. Cardiac monitoring and intravenous access are desirable, if available, particularly if the victim has suffered loss of consciousness or complains of chest pain or difficulty breathing.

For the more seriously injured victim, the airway should be assessed and protected, if necessary. Cardiopulmonary resuscitation, if indicated, should be instituted with appropriate advanced cardiac life support (ACLS) protocols being followed. Routine ACLS drugs may be used as normally indicated by the patient's condition. Spinal immobilization should be done for the unconscious patient or one who has suffered a fall or been thrown in the incident.

Assessing the blood pressure may be difficult, as some victims have intense vascular spasm with cool, nearly pulseless extremities. Occasionally, the blood pressure will be found to be elevated due to vascular constriction. This will usually resolve on its own without the need for medication or other intervention. The lower extremities and occasionally the upper extremities may appear mottled, pulseless, and cool as a result of vascular spasm or sympathetic nervous system instability. This, too, usually resolves in a matter of hours, although there may be permanent paresis and paresthesia in some patients.

Intravenous fluid should be lactated Ringer's or normal saline. Normally, fluid restriction is preferred for these patients, especially those who are in cardiac arrest or who have blunt injuries to the head, in order to prevent cerebral edema. However, if there are signs that shock is due to blunt injury, multiple major fractures, or blood loss, fluid resuscitation should be more vigorous.

Physical assessment should also include a brief evaluation of the mental status of the victim and a search for burns, fractures, and dislocations. Victims should be transported to a hospital for further treatment, if necessary, and evaluation.

II. EMERGENCY DEPARTMENT CARE

A. STABILIZATION

Immediate care should address patency and protection of the airway and institution of cardiac (ACLS) protocols if indicated by the victim's presentation. Intravenous access, if not already obtained by the EMS personnel, is indicated in the more severely injured or unconscious victim.

B. EVALUATION AND TREATMENT

It is helpful to obtain a history, if it is available, of the incident. In addition, a history of the patient's health status, including allergies, medications, and concurrent illnesses, can be helpful in guiding further care after resuscitation.

As with all trauma patients, it is essential that the patient be undressed in order to facilitate a complete physical evaluation. Not only are the vital signs essential, but the physician should take note of the mental status of the patient and note it on the chart. Since many victims will have been hit during a thunderstorm and will be wet, the patient should also be evaluated for hypothermia and treated appropriately.

Victims of lightning injury who present to an emergency department need to be evaluated by the emergency physician for cardiac damage, including arrhythmias; neurological damage, including intracranial and spinal cord injury; burns, including a screen for myoglobinuria if the burns are extensive; tympanic membrane rupture and hearing loss; injuries to the musculoskeletal system, including fractures, dislocations, and spinal trauma; and ophthalmic injury.

If the patient is still in cardiac arrest by the time they reach the emergency department, cardiopulmonary resuscitation may be continued until it is judged that recovery is unlikely. The postcardiac arrest and resuscitation patient who recovers cardiac function and a blood pressure should be treated as if they have had a myocardial infarction, or at least myocardial damage, with appropriate monitoring for arrhythmias and serial electrocardiograms and cardiac enzymes. The drug regimen for these patients for arrhythmias is the same as in standard cardiac care. Electrocardiographic changes may take several weeks to months to resolve.

It is probably wise to obtain an electrocardiogram even in the patient who has not had a cardiac arrest, since they may occasionally show ST segment changes and arrhythmias. If the patient is otherwise alert and not complaining of chest pain, cardiac monitoring may not be necessary.

Severe vascular spasm of the extremities may be present in up to two thirds of victims, with cold, pulseless, mottled extremities making it difficult to obtain an accurate blood pressure. A Doppler may need to be used to measure the blood pressure. Fluid restriction should be the rule in most of these patients in order to decrease the amount of cerebral edema that they may suffer. However, if there is evidence of true shock, the physician should rule out spinal cord injury and spinal shock. In addition, hypovolemic shock should be ruled out or treated with vigorous fluid resuscitation.

Vascular spasm affects the lower extremities nearly twice as often as the upper extremities and is probably a result of sympathetic nervous system instability as well as vascular spasm. While it usually clears within a few hours, the victim should nevertheless be observed for any untoward complications, such as compartment syndrome or evolving neurologic damage secondary to cord ischemia from spinal artery spasm, with frequent neurovascular checks.

Frequently, the victim will have suffered unconsciousness, even if only temporarily, may be combative and confused as his mental state continues to clear, and will be amnesic for the event and often for the events of the next few days, similar to the victim of electroconvulsive shock therapy for depression. The victim who does not continue to clear neurologically must be assessed for intracranial injury, including intracranial hemorrhage, cerebral contusion, and skull fracture, which have all been reported. Computerized tomography or nuclear magnetic resonance scanning is indicated in these patients.

The burns that are seen with lightning injury have already been discussed in Chapters 5 and 6. As noted, they are generally superficial and require little but supportive care. The deep burns that are common with man-made high-voltage electrical injuries are uncommon with lightning, but, if they occur, should be treated as high-voltage burns usually are — with fluid loading, alkalinization of the urine, osmotic diuresis, and fasciotomy as indicated. Lightning injuries seldom need this aggressive care and burns are generally the least of all the problems that may be seen with lightning victims.

Tympanic rupture is common with lightning victims, although the physician generally does not know to look for it initially in most cases. In addition to tympanic membrane rupture, ossicular disruption may occur. The patient needs referral to a qualified otolaryngologist for evaluation and care, although operative intervention is usually delayed until after the edema and inflammation of the acute injury resolve. Otorrhea or hemotympanum may indicate basilar skull fracture.

While fractures and dislocations have been reported with lightning injuries, they are relatively uncommon unless the victim has been thrown a distance. Nevertheless, the secondary survey of the patient after they have been stabilized should include a search for them. Particularly dangerous are spinal injuries. If there is any evidence that the patient has been thrown or fallen, the cervical spine should be evaluated for damage, and cervical immobilization should continue until it can be ruled out. This is particularly important in the unconscious or intoxicated patient who cannot give a history or cooperate with the physical examination. In the conscious, alert patient who is sober and who has had no loss of consciousness, spinal injury usually can be easily ruled out clinically without radiography.

The abdomen should be evaluated for blunt trauma, although it is uncommon. The absence of bowel sounds may indicate only a simple ileus or may be more ominous and indicate intraabdominal injury. Since gastric irritation may occur in the more seriously injured patient, histamine antagonists and antacids may be indicated as well as nasogastric suction. Peritoneal lavage or abdominal scanning may be indicated if the patient continues to show signs of shock or has other evidence of intraabdominal injury.

Sometime during the initial examination but after the patient has been stabilized, the eyes should be evaluated for any damage, including cataract formation. It is useful, if the patient can cooperate, to obtain a visual acuity so that any deterioration over the next few days can be documented.

Tetanus prophylaxis should be given if indicated by history and physical examination. Antibiotics need not be given unless there are signs of significant open injuries, violation of the dura, or intraabdominal injuries.

C. DISPOSITION

Minimally or moderately injured patients usually continue to improve dramatically over the first few hours. The minimally injured patient will probably only need overnight observation or may even be discharged to a responsible family member if the physician judges this to be appropriate after evaluation. The moderately injured patient may need hospitalization while their mental status improves and for further evaluation and perhaps rehabilitation planning for their injuries. Obviously, the most seriously injured victims may need intensive care, with extensive monitoring and often mechanical ventilation, antiarrhythmic medication, and Swan-Ganz catheterization.

D. LABORATORY AND RADIOLOGIC EXAMINATIONS

For the minimally injured victim, a thorough physical examination, an electrocardiogram, and appropriate referral for follow-up may be all that is indicated. However, based on the physician's findings, other tests may also be appropriate.

For more seriously injured patients, a complete blood count, electrocardiogram, cardiac enzymes, and urinalysis for myoglobin are indicated along with any other tests that are specifically indicated by the patient's physical findings. The most seriously ill patients will obviously need more aggressive laboratory examination and monitoring, including arterial blood gases if they have suffered a cardiac arrest or are on a mechanical ventilator, electrolytes, and kidney function tests such as blood urea nitrogen (BUN) and creatinine for use as a baseline. Serial cardiac isoenzymes and electrocardiograms are probably indicated for these patients.

An X-ray of the chest may be helpful in the moderately or severely injured patient. Cervical spine films should be ordered for anyone who has had a loss of consciousness, a history of being thrown, cranial burns, contusions, or change in mentation. Other films may be indicated by the patient's history and physical examination. If there is evidence of intracranial injury or edema, computerized tomography or nuclear magnetic resonance scanning are indicated, and intracranial pressure monitoring may be helpful. Obviously, operable causes of intracranial injury require operative intervention, depending on the general expectation for the survival of the patient.

An electrocardiogram is necessary for all patients due to the relatively high incidence of cardiac injuries with lightning stroke.

III. INTENSIVE CARE MANAGEMENT

R. P. F. Parkes
(with a contribution by M. J. Eadie)

A. INTRODUCTION

Following initial assessment and resuscitation of a patient suffering from lightning strike, therapy should be directed toward inpatient care. Patients who are conscious on presentation and who have no evidence of severe burns, respiratory failure, or cardiac disease may be successfully managed in a center with limited facilities. All patients should receive at least 24 h of electrocardiographic (ECG) monitoring attended by medical and nursing staff skilled in the interpretation of arrhythmias and cardiopulmonary resuscitation (CPR). Multisystem pathology, however, may require referral to a general intensive care unit (ICU). Table 1 lists the human and technical resources required for the successful management of severe lightning strike. Transfer to a regional referral center is recommended for the management of life-threatening multisystem disease, for long-term (>48 h) intermittent positive pressure ventilation (IPPV), renal dialysis, or the evaluation and management of persistent coma. Severe cardiac failure or the presence of significant arrhythmias should prompt referral to a center with expertise in cardiology.

Imagine your predicament, however, when asked to manage a patient suffering the effects of lightning strike. After reading the contributions from the other authors of this book, your accident and emergency colleagues have elegantly resuscitated the patient and now seek to refer him or her to you for ongoing care. You remember that your old friend, Dr. X, knew a bit about lightning (still, his experience must be limited; lightning only strikes once in the same place!). This review aims to present the features of lightning strike in a manner that will assist the clinician in intensive care practice. No attempt will be made to discuss burns, ocular, or ear, nose, and throat injuries.

B. PUBLISHED EXPERIENCE WITH LIGHTNING INJURY

Lightning injury is uncommon. Occasionally, a number of individuals will be affected;[1] in general, however, the literature is restricted to individual reports or cumulative reviews. While frequently reported events infer a significant clinical problem, the retrospective nature of such reports and the lack of standardized reporting do not necessarily assist with individual patient management. Intensive care is a relatively new specialty. Although earlier reports elegantly describe the natural history of lightning strike, any therapeutic regimen in which CPR and IPPV are not available is difficult to relate to current intensive care practice. For this reason, this discussion will be largely restricted to cases reported after 1960,[2] when CPR was first advocated. The principal clinical syndromes of relevance to intensive care are listed in Table 2.[3-35]

TABLE 1
Human and Physical Resources Required for the
Management of Severe Lightning Injury

An intensive care unit with:
   24-h medical and nursing staff
   One-to-one nurse/patient ratio
   ECG monitoring
   Cardioversion
   Facilities for ventilation

A hospital with:
   24-h laboratory service
   24-h radiology service
   (including CT scanning)
      Access to specialist services:
         Orthopedic surgery
         Neurosurgery
         ENT surgery
         Ophthalmology
         General surgery
         Burns surgery
         Cardiology

C. INTENSIVE CARE MANAGEMENT

1. The Cardiovascular System

Resuscitation commences with the stabilization of airway, breathing, and circulation.[36] ECG monitoring should be instituted as soon as possible and arrhythmias treated. Individual experience has not shown a clear pattern of arrhythmias after lightning strike. Although bystander CPR is usually commenced in the absence of a palpable peripheral pulse, the administration of CPR may not necessarily imply the presence of cardiac arrest. In 17 patients reported as receiving CPR in recent literature,[2-4,6-8,11,13,20,22,25-27] CPR was initiated in 5 instances where no arrhythmia was present.[11,13,22,26,27] Although bystander overenthusiasm may be one reason for this (in one case, the person initiating resuscitation was a medical student!), apnea, rather than an arrythmia, may be the indication for CPR (see Section III.C.3 below).

In assessing the circulation, the complexity of lightning strike should be borne in mind. Burns, trauma, blast injuries, and hypothermia may complicate the electrical injury. Therefore, in addition to the diagnosis and treatment of arrhythmias, a search should be made for other causes of circulatory collapse. In the presence of sinus rhythm, circulatory collapse may be due to hypovolemia, myocardial injury (including myocardial contusion), and cardiac tamponade. With regard to cardiac tamponade, the classical signs of elevated venous pressure, Kussmaul's sign, paradoxical pulse, and a quiet precordium may not always be present, particularly in a ventilated patient; echocardiography should be performed if possible. This will give additional information regarding focal and global myocardial function. In most cases, fluid administration is guided by the assessment of pulse, blood pressure, skin perfusion, urine output, and central venous pressure. Addition information may be gained after placement of a pulmonary artery (Swan Ganz) catheter. The principal indications for insertion are:

1.   To elucidate the differential diagnosis of pulmonary edema (elevated pulmonary venous pressure vs. the adult respiratory distress syndrome)
2.   To allow greater precision in fluid resuscitation
3.   To aid in the diagnosis of cardiac tamponade
4.   To aid in the differentiation between an acquired ventricular septal defect and mitral papillary muscle rupture.

TABLE 2
Common Clinical Events in Lightning Strike

	Ref.
Cardiovascular	
Inferior myocardial infarction	3,4,6,16,18,26–28
Anterior myocardial infarction	14,18,23,28
Ventricular fibrillation	3,4,6.8,20,22,27
Ventricular asystole	2,6,25
Need for cardiopulmonary resuscitation	2–4,6–8,11,13,20,22,25–27
Pulmonary	
Diffuse pulmonary infiltrates	2,3,6,8,11,13–15,22,23,25
Bronchospasm	6
Need for IPPV	2,3,6,8,11–14,15,26,31
Central nervous system	
Motor paralysis	21,23,26,28,33
Mononeuritis	10,26,30
Brain death	3,6,22,31
Persisting cerebral damage	8,11,22,26,27
Cerebral trauma	3,6,7,13,22,26,31,32,34
Paraplegia	24
Gastrointestinal system	
Acute abdomen	8,22
Gastrointestinal hemorrhage	10
Acute gastric dilatation	6,25
Chronic abdominal pain	5
Renal system	
Myoglobinuria	4,5,8,20,35
Hemoglobinuria	4,8,20
Miscellaneous	
DIC	3
Hypothermia	2,6,8,25
Focal cutaneous necrosis	12
Hypertension, tachycardia	4,7,11,23

While normal sinus rhythm and consciousness on presentation imply a good prognosis, ECG abnormalities of myocardial damage have been frequently reported. Inferior myocardial infarction[3,4,6,16,26-28] has been reported more frequently than anterior infarction.[14,18,23,28] If myocardial infarction occurs, circulatory problems appear to be uncommon in the absence of other pathology. In general, therefore, the expectant management of a patient with myocardial function is adequate. Although thrombolytic therapy after transmural myocardial infarction has been demonstrated to reduce mortality,[37] lightning strike is accompanied by a high incidence of associated trauma and prolonged CPR. For this reason, thrombolytic agents should be used with caution. Particular attention should be given to the provision of adequate analgesia, as pain typical of myocardial ischemia occurs.[19]

2. The Respiratory System

Assessment of the respiratory system should commence with an evaluation of the patient's airway and ventilation and examination for pulmonary edema, a flail segment, and aspiration pneumonitis. A chest X-ray should be taken soon after admission and arterial blood gases should be sampled if clinically indicated.

TABLE 3
Differential Diagnosis of Bilateral Pulmonary Infiltrates
Appearing within 24 h of Admission for Lightning Strike

Cardiogenic pulmonary edema
Aspiration pneumonitis
Pulmonary contusion
Blast injury
Thermal injury
"Neurogenic" pulmonary edema
Preexisting pulmonary disease

The need for positive pressure ventilation was identified in 10 case reports.[2,3,6,8,11-14,15,26,31] Although many patients were intubated as part of the process of CPR or for frank respiratory failure, IPPV was frequently instituted as an aid to the management of persistent coma. The importance of an adequate airway cannot be overemphasized. If the patient has a depressed gag or cough reflex and can tolerate a Guedel airway, an endotracheal tube should be inserted and the patient ventilated to protect the airway, maintain oxygenation, and avoid the deleterious effects of hypercapnia. Arterial hypoxemia may not necessarily indicate the need for intubation and ventilation in a conscious, lucid patient. For example, left ventricular failure may be associated with significant hypoxemia, but may respond to conservative measures such as the administration of diuretics and oxygen by mask. Patients with pulmonary and chest wall trauma may not require IPPV if pain is relieved, the patient remains lucid, and cough is effective.

Although myocardial infarction is common, the presence of bilateral pulmonary infiltrates may not necessarily be due to left ventricular failure. Other insults may produce a similar radiological picture (Table 3). To elucidate this, gram stain and bacteriological assessment of sputum, echocardiography, and flow-directed pulmonary artery (Swan-Ganz) catheterization may be indicated. Therapy for respiratory failure includes treatment of the underlying cause (LVF, infection) and the general medical and nursing care of a patient on a ventilator.[38] This will not be reviewed here.

3. Central Nervous System
a. Assessment
As soon as possible, a rapid assessment of neurological function should be made. In addition to an assessment of conscious state, the Glasgow coma score (GCS) should be documented and a search made for focal neurological signs.

External signs of head trauma have been frequently reported.[3,6,7,13,22,26,31,32] Although focal intracranial pathology is uncommon, extradural, subdural, and intracerebral hematomata[7,13,34] have been reported. Computerized axial tomography (CAT) scanning should be performed in cases of persistent coma, particularly when an initially conscious patient becomes comatose,[7] when signs of external head trauma are present, or when focal neurological signs are observed.

Ravitch et al.[2] and Taussig[21] advocated prolonged CPR after cases of lightning strike, noting recovery of consciousness and mentation after prolonged anoxia. However, the literature reveals that the morbidity and mortality are high. A critical review by Cooper[39] demonstrated a poor prognosis after the onset of ventricular fibrillation. In nine reports of ventricular fibrillation[3,4,6,8,20,22,27] and three reports of asystole,[2,6,25] brain death occurred in four cases.[3,6,22,31] Persisting neurological deficits were observed in a further five and included loss of short-term memory,[8] ataxia,[22] recurrent seizures,[11] and alterations in personality.[20,26,27] Although apparent recovery after prolonged anoxia has occurred,[2,19,25] a prospective study with standardized criteria for assessment of neurologic function is required to accurately describe the natural history of cerebral damage following lightning strike.

Keraunoparalysis,[33] characterized by the triad of motor paralysis, anesthesia and vasomotor disturbance, may be encountered during initial assessment.[21,23,26,28,34] Typically, the pulse in an affected limb is absent. The pathophysiology is imperfectly understood, but may be due to spasm of the vasa vasorum. Paralysis, however, is transient; full recovery of motor and sensory function usually occurs within 1 to 2 d.

Spinal cord injury has been reported;[24] a diagnosis of keraunoparalysis should only be made after structural spinal cord injury has been excluded. In complete cord transection, impaired anal reflexes and autonomic disturbance such as priapism and urinary retention are observed. These events are not described in keraunoparalysis. A symmetrical motor neuropathy of both lower limbs has also been described.[26]

Coma as a presenting sign is frequently reported; its duration is variable. IPPV is therefore indicated to protect the airway and to assist in the control of intracranial pressure (ICP). In general, the arterial PCO_2 should be maintained at approximately 25 to 30 mmHg. Fluid restriction, steroids, diuretics, barbiturates, calcium channel blockers, lignocaine, phenytoin, and osmotic agents have all been used to minimize cerebral damage.[40] ICP monitoring is frequently used in a number of institutions.

Brain death may occur after lightning strike. The diagnosis may be clouded by hypothermia,[2,6,8,25] keraunoparalysis, and damage to the vestibular system (Chapter 5). Keraunoparalysis may delay, but will not prevent a diagnosis of brain death, as it rarely involves the face and seldom, if ever, persists after 48 h. The diagnosis of brain death, therefore, may be made if brain stem reflexes are absent after careful examination on two occasions, if an appropriate clinical situation exists, and if metabolic, pharmacologic, or other causes of coma are excluded.[41]

b. Management (Contributed by M. J. Eadie)

When cardiac arrest follows lightning strike, the early institution of CPR may be life saving. Death is unlikely in the absence of cardiac arrest[39] and there is published evidence that the institution of CPR may permit the survival of patients judged clinically dead by conventional criteria.[2,21] The other acute neurological effects of lightning injury are likely to resolve spontaneously within a relatively short period. There do not seem to be published data suggesting that active intervention (apart from resuscitation) improves the prognosis in the majority of instances of lightning injury to the central nervous system

The rare delayed neurological sequelae of lightning strike appear to involve a number of different pathogenic mechanisms, although some are not elucidated. The presence of intracranial bleeding can now be established by CT head scanning and, if necessary, appropriate steps can be taken to reduce intracranial pressure (e.g., high-dose glucocorticoids, intravenous osmotically active cerebral dehydrating agents), and/or surgical evacuation of a hematoma if it constitutes a significant mass lesion and is situated in an accessible site. Any residual neurological deficit is managed in the usual way, e.g., physiotherapy, speech therapy, as indicated.

4. Gastrointestinal System

Acute gastric dilatation[6,25] and stress erosions have been described.[10] In all patients requiring IPPV, the stomach should be decompressed with a nasogastric tube and prophylaxis against stress ulceration commenced. Antacids and histamine (H2 receptor) antagonists are effective in preventing stress ulceration. However, evidence suggests that sucralfate conveys effective protection with a lower incidence of hospital-acquired pneumonia.[42]

A continued search for evidence of intraabdominal pathology is vital. The interpretation of signs is difficult in the setting of a sedated, ventilated patient. Abdominal ultrasound, CAT scanning, radioisotope scanning of the abdomen and, in selected cases, "blind" laparotomy may be necessary to reveal the source of hemorrhage or sepsis.[43,44]

5. Renal System

Both myoglobinuria[4,5,8,20,35] and hemoglobinuria[4,8,20] have been recorded following lightning strike. Unfortunately, their severity is difficult to estimate from published reports. Modest amounts of myoglobin or acid hematein are rapidly excreted by the kidney; however, massive amounts may cause acute renal failure. Excretion of myoglobin is enhanced by increasing urine volume and the maintenance of an alkaline urine. The use of mannitol and intravenous sodium bicarbonate is protective.[45] However, increased urinary losses must be replaced and renal perfusion maintained. Attention should also be directed toward the provision of adequate urinary drainage, the prevention of urinary tract infection, and maintenance of adequate renal perfusion.

6. Miscellaneous
a. Hypothermia

Hypothermia has been recorded.[2,6,8,25] Prevention of further heat loss by gentle warming and adequate humidification of inspired gases will frequently result in restoration of normal body temperature. Surface rewarming is more rapid, but may result in hypotension due to cutaneous vasodilatation. Internal rewarming using an extracorporeal circulation, irrigation of the peritoneum or mediastinum, may (rarely) be required.[46] The relative rarity of hypothermia as a clinical entity casts doubt on the postulate that metabolic rate falls dramatically.[21,47]

b. Disseminated Intravascular Coagulation

Disseminated intravascular coagulation has been reported following prolonged hypoxia.[3] In addition, the syndrome may result from burns, sepsis, fat embolism, and, in the case of a female patient, a missed abortion.

c. Hyperadrenergic State

A "hyperadrenergic state", characterized by the presence of hypertension and tachycardia, has been reported.[4,7,11,23] While this may be a specific feature of lightning stroke, a similar clinical picture is frequently encountered in critically ill patients; evaluation of the patient for left ventricular failure, pain, sepsis, hypovolemia, or preexisting hypertension should be undertaken. While β-blockers have been advocated for this condition, they are contraindicated in patients with cardiac failure or airway obstruction.

d. Care of the Family

The patient's family may have witnessed both the violence of the lightning strike and the apparent violence of subsequent resuscitation and urgent evacuation. In addition to a simple explanation of the nature of the injury and the proposed therapy, they will need reassurance that, at least, everything possible is being done. It is important to explain that "everything possible" may not be enough, i.e., that the patient may die. A statement that "everything will be all right" may lead relatives down an unrealistic path. If everything is *not* all right, that path may end in the destruction of the family, refusal to accept that therapy is pointless, and anger directed at the ICU team. Such anger is typically expressed in litigation.

IV. INPATIENT MANAGEMENT AND FOLLOW-UP

A. POST-INTENSIVE CARE ASSESSMENT

Following discharge from the ICU or CCU, the physician has an active role to play. Transfer should be accompanied by an early and thorough physical examination. The use of sedative, analgesic, and relaxant drugs used in the ICU may mask focal neurological signs.

B. NEUROLOGICAL REHABILITATION

In the event of evidence of cerebral damage, a skilled team is required to assess, supervise, and maximize the patient's recovery, and referral to a rehabilitation unit is essential.

In addition to diffuse and focal cerebral damage, a mononeuritis has been reported[10,26,30] with impaired nerve conduction.[26] While the prognosis appears good, its presence may have medicolegal implications for a patient wishing to document his or her level of disability.

Personality changes may occur as a result of cerebral anoxia, the effects of injury, bereavement, and hospitalization. In a study of affected children, Dollinger et al.[48] described a high incidence of fears, somatic complaints, and sleep disturbance. Furthermore, a sense of guilt is particularly common in individuals who survive a disaster; all victims should be counseled to treat emotional disturbance.

C. CARDIAC REHABILITATION AND COUNSELING

ECG abnormalities are said to resolve within 12 months (Chapter 5, q.v.). However, the risk of chronic cardiac disease following lightning strike is unknown. Furthermore, some patients with an abnormal ECG will have severe preexisting cardiac disease. Ongoing assessment of cardiac function should continue, therefore, for at least 12 months. Arrhythmias, angina, or cardiac failure should prompt referral for expert cardiac assessment of cardiac anatomy and function.

Truly elective surgery should probably be avoided for 6 months. Following myocardial infarction, the incidence of intraoperative myocardial infarction is considerably increased; this risk declines to approximately 15% at 6 months.[49]

Pregnancy aggravates preexisting cardiac disease. Although there are no published data, it would seem prudent to counsel women of child-bearing age who have suffered myocardial damage as a result of lightning strike to avoid conception for a period of 12 months.

In addition to the acute gastric dilatation and abdominal visceral injury described above, chronic abdominal pain has been described.[5] Its nature is poorly understood; symptomatic treatment has been employed with limited success.

D. CONCLUSIONS

Lightning strike poses a significant threat to life. In the event of severe, multisystem disease, shock, or respiratory failure, admission to an ICU with appropriate clinical and laboratory facilities is essential. The role of the intensive care specialist in such a situation is fourfold: (1) to provide life support, (2) to ensure that other diseases which may mimic lightning injury are excluded, (3) to arrange appropriate specialist referral, and (4) to care for the patient's family. Adequate follow-up is an equally important part of care. An integrated team approach will ensure that the patient's recovery is maximized.

REFERENCES

1. **Arden, G. P., Harrison, S. H., Lister, J., and Maudsley, R. H.,** Lightning injury at Ascot, *Br. Med. J.,* 1, 1450, 1956.
2. **Ravitch, M. M., Lane, R., Safar, P., Steichen, F. M., and Knowles, P.,** Lightning stroke, *N. Engl. J. Med.,* 264, 36, 1961.
3. **Ekoe, J. M., Cunningham, M., Jaques, O., Balague, F., Baumann, R. P., Humair, L., and de Torrente, A.,** Disseminated intravascular coagulation and acute myocardial necrosis caused by lightning, *Intens. Care. Med.,* 11, 160, 1985.
4. **Yost, J. W. and Holmes, F. F.,** Myoglobinuria following lightning stroke, *JAMA,* 228, 1147, 1974.

5. **Akahane, T. and Okishio, R.,** Lightning injury: report of two cases, *Burns,* 10, 45, 1980.
6. **Hanson, L. C. and McIlwraith, G. R.,** Lightning injury: two case histories and a review of management, *Br. Med. J.,* 4, 271, 1973.
7. **Morgan, Z. V., Headley, R. N., Alexander, E. A., and Sawyer, C. G.,** Atrial fibrillation and epidural hematoma associated with lightning stroke, *N. Engl. J. Med.,* 259, 956, 1958.
8. **Smith, J.,** Lightning injuries, *J. Emerg. Nurs.,* 9(5), 248, 1983.
9. **Dowling, J., Byrne, K., Barry, O. C. D., Long, J. P., and Lennon, F.,** Lightning injury, *Ir. Med. J.,* 77, 250, 1984.
10. **Amy, B. W., McManus, W. F., Goodwin, C. W., and Pruitt, B. A.,** Lightning injury with survival in five patients, *JAMA,* 253, 243, 1985.
11. **McCrady, V. L. and Kahn, M.,** Lightning burns, *West. J. Med.,* 134, 215, 1981.
12. **Ehsan, M., Waxman, J., and Finley, J. M.,** Delayed gangrene after lightning strike, *AFP,* 24, 117, 1981.
13. **Stanley, L. D. and Suss, R. A.,** Intracerebral haematoma secondary to lightning stroke: case report and review of the literature, *Neurosurgery,* 16, 686, 1985.
14. **Kleiner, J. P. and Wilkin, J. H.,** Cardiac effects of lightning stroke, *JAMA,* 240, 2757, 1978.
15. **Moulson, A. M.,** Blast injury of the lungs due to lightning, *Br. Med. J.,* 289, 1270, 1984.
16. **Subramanian, N., Somasundram, B., and Periasamy, J. K.,** Cardiac injury due to lightning — report of a survivor, *Ind. Heart J.,* 37, 72, 1985.
17. **Zeana, C. D.,** Acute transient myocardial ischemia after lightning injury, *Int. J. Cardiol.,* 5, 207, 1984.
18. **Jackson, S. H. D.,** Lightning and the heart, *Br. Heart J.,* 43, 454, 1980.
19. **Sinha, A. K.,** Lightning induced myocardial injury — a case report with management, *Angiology,* 36(5), 327, 1985.
20. **Apfelberg, D. B. et al.,** Pathophysiology of treatment of lightning injuries, *J. Trauma,* 14(6), 453, 1974.
21. **Taussig, H. A.,** "Death" from lightning — and the possibility of living again, *Ann. Int. Med.,* 68(6), 1345, 1968.
22. **Krob, M. J. et al.,** Lightning injuries: a multisystem trauma, *J. Iowa Med. Soc.,* 73(6), 221, 1983.
23. **Peters, W. J.,** Lightning injury, *Can. Med. Assoc. J.,* 128, 148, 1983.
24. **Sharma, M. and Smith, A.,** Paraplegia as a result of lightning injury, *Br. Med. J.,* November, 1464, 1978.
25. **Morikawa, S. et al.,** Successful resuscitation after "death" from lightning, *Anesthesiology,* 21, 223, 1960.
26. **Moran, K. T. et al.,** Lightning injury, physics, pathophysiology and clinical features, *Ir. Med. J.,* 79(5), 120, 1986.
27. **Moran, K. T. et al.,** Electric and lightning induced cardiac arrest reversed by prompt cardiopulmonary resuscitation (lett.), *JAMA,* 255(16), 2157, 1986b.
28. **Kleinot, S. et al.,** The cardiac effects of lightning injury, *S. Afr. Med. J.,* 40, 1141, 1966.
29. **Kristensen, S. et al.,** Lightning induced acoustic rupture of the tympanic membrane (a report of two cases), *J. Laryngol., Otol.,* 99, 711, 1985.
30. **Weiss, K. S.,** Otological lightning bolts, *Am. J. Otol.,* 1, 334, 1980.
31. **Mann, H., et al.,** CT of lightning injury, *Am. J. Neuroradiol.,* 4, 976, 1983.
32. **Poulsen, P. and Knudstrup, P.,** Lightning causing inner ear damage and intracranial haematoma, *J. Laryngol. Otol.,* 100, 1067, 1986.
33. **ten Duis, H. J. et al.,** Keraunoparalysis, a "specific" lightning injury, *Burns,* 12(1), 54, 1985.
34. **Strasser, E. J. et al.,** Lightning injuries, *J. Trauma,* 17, 315, 1977.
35. **Yost, J. W. et al.,** Myoglobinuria following lightning stroke, *JAMA,* 228, 1147, 1974.
36. Standards and guidelines for cardiopulmonary resuscitation (CPR) and emergency cardiac care (ECC), *JAMA,* 255, 2905, 1986.
37. ISIS 2 (2nd Int. Study Infarct Survival) collaborative group, A randomised trial of intravenous streptokinase, oral aspirin, both, or neither among 17,187 cases of suspected acute myocardial infarction: ISIS 2, *Lancet,* 2, 349, 1988.
38. **Downs, J. B. and Stock, M. C.,** *Current Therapy in Critical Care Medicine,* Parillo, J. E., Ed., B. C. Decker, 1987, 19.
39. **Cooper, M. A.,** Lightning injuries: prognostic signs for death, *Ann. Emerg. Med.,* 9, 134, 1980.
40. **Oh, T. E.,** *Intensive Care Manual,* 2nd ed., Butterworths, Sydney, 1985, chap. 36.
41. **Oh, T. E.,** *Intensive Care Manual,* 2nd ed., Butterworths, Sydney, 1985, chap. 37.
42. **Bresalier, R. S., Grendall, J. H., Cello, J. P., and Meyre, A. A.,** Sucralfate suspension versus titrated antacid for the prevention of acute stress-related gastrointestinal haemorrhage in critically ill patients, *Am. J. Med.,* 83(Suppl. 3B), 110, 1987.
43. **Snyder, S. K. and Hahn, H. H.,** Diagnosis and treatment of intraabdominal abscess in critically ill patients, *Surg. Clin. North Am.,* 62, 229, 1982.
44. **Polk, H. C. and Shields, C. L.,** Remote organ failure: a valid sign of intraabdominal infection, *Surgery,* 81, 310, 1977.

45. **Eneas, J. F., Schoenfield, P. Y., and Humphreys, M. H.,** The effect of infusion of mannitol-sodium bicarbonate on the clinical course of myoglobinuria, *Arch. Int. Med.,* 139, 801, 1979.
46. **Reed, G. and Knochel, J. P.,** Hypothermia, in *Current Therapy in Critical Care Medicine,* Parillo, J. E., Ed., B. C. Decker, 1987, 324.
47. **Bartholome, C. W. et al.,** Cutaneous manifestations of lightning injury, *Arch. Dermatol,* 111, 1466, 1975.
48. **Dollinger, S. J., O'Donnell, J. P., and Staley, A. A.,** Lightning strike disaster: effects on fears and worries, *J. Consult. Clin. Psychol.,* 52, 1028, 1984.
49. **Weitz, H. W. and Goldman, I.,** Non cardiac surgery in the patient with heart disease, *Med. Clin. North Am.,* 71(3), 413, 1987.

V. SPECIAL ASPECTS OF OCULAR MANAGEMENT

F. Fraunfelder and M. Meyer

A. EMERGENCY CARE

Contrary to the popular belief that being struck by lightning is nearly always fatal, many more survive than die. Sudden death in lightning injuries is the result of paralysis of the respiratory center, apnea, ventricular fibrillation, or cardiac arrest.

1. Aggressive Resuscitation

Artificial resuscitative measures should be started early and continued almost indefinitely after lightning injuries. Dilated or nonreactive pupils are an unreliable indicator of severe brain-stem hypoxia in a patient injured by lightning. Pupillary responses should never be used as a criterion to withhold or discontinue aggressive resuscitative measures in these patients.[1]

2. Increased Intracranial Pressure

Treatment of increased intracranial pressure following lightning injuries includes hyperventilation, steroids, and hyperosmolar agents. The benefits of these treatments can be assessed by monitoring the patient's intracranial pressure.[2]

B. PRIMARY CARE

While the best treatment for ocular injuries from lightning is prevention, actual treatment is supportive. It is aimed at preventing infection and tissue loss.

1. Tetanus Prophylaxis

Prophylactic treatment of a major burn wound should include an injection of 0.5 ml of adsorbed tetanus toxoid to all patients who have not had a booster within the past year. In nonvaccinated subjects, immunization will be completed by two further injections, at 4 to 6 weeks and then at 6 months.

2. Cleansing and Debridement of the Wound

The lids may have typical cutaneous burn injuries. Depending on the severity, superficial to deep burns leading to sloughing may occur. The burned areas should be kept clean by applying warm, wet sterile gauze impregnated with antibiotics such as gentamicin, and the necrotic tissue should be gently debrided.[3]

Corneal injuries are the most common immediate ocular findings in lightning strikes, and generally consist of epithelial layer lesions and deep opacities that may require several weeks to resolve.[4] Corneal exposure may be avoided by patching and applying moist compresses or a moisture chamber. Occasionally, the use of a soft contact lens may be necessary.

C. INTERMEDIARY CARE

The immediate management of acute electrical injuries of the eye is the preservation of eyelid structure and motility, the maintenance of conjunctival fornices, and the provision of an adequate cover for the anterior segment of the eye. Intraocular inflammation should be carefully controlled by the judicious use of corticosteroids and mydriatics. There is no proven therapy for retinopathy associated with severe electrical burns; however, systemic corticosteroids might theoretically help preserve retinal structure and function if the patient's general condition does not contraindicate the use of such drugs in high doses. Long-term sequelae, such as cataract formation, are more amenable to treatment, and surgery for this condition is usually uneventful. Where there has been severe loss of central vision, low visual aids (magnification devices) may be of some help in improving the patient's reading capability.

1. Antimicrobial Therapy

While dead tissue remains, bacterial activity is heightened; while the wound remains open, bacterial invasion may occur. *Pseudomonas aeruginosa* and *Staphylococcus aureus* are the predominant organisms in the majority of significant burn wound infections; streptococci and *Proteus* are less frequent.

Systemic antibiotics should be used as indicated to treat or prevent infection secondary to either lightning or electrical injury. Oral oxytetracycline or parenteral gentamicin or potassium penicillin G may be administered. The usual daily dosage of gentamicin is 3 mg/kg given i.v. or i.m. in three divided doses. Ocular measures to keep burned eyelids free of infection may include use of polymyxin B wet applications.

2. Temporary Corneal Grafts

Allografts or porcine xenografts may be used to alleviate pain, prevent secondary infection, and hasten the healing process of corneal injury. If possible, autografts should be used for permanent wound closure.

3. Additional Ocular Repairs

Severe corneal involvement with impending corneal perforation secondary to thermal injuries may require penetrating keratoplasty. When possible, tarsorrhaphy should be performed to protect the graft and globe.[5] Between 75 and 80% of electrical cataracts will progress to the point where lens extraction is required.[6,7]

4. Cycloplegics and Corticosteroids

Iridocyclitis may develop, depending on the degree of lightning injury. Anterior uveitis may be treated by application of 1 to 2% atropine four times daily.[8] Early and constant pupillary dilatation lessens the likelihood of synechias. For treatment of severe uveitis, one drop of 0.1% dexamethasone two to four times daily may be added to the mydriatic regimen.

D. RECONSTRUCTIVE CARE

Treatment of survivors of lightning injury may also include reconstructive care when clinical observation indicates no improvement. Surgical procedures are performed to restore the eye as nearly as possible to its original state.

1. Skin Grafts for Eyelids

Lightning burns are generally more superficial than those caused by high-voltage alternating current. Conservative management is indicated, and skin grafting is seldom necessary for achieving burn wound closure of the eyelids; however, if so, the lids may require split- or full-thickness grafts and nasal cartilage to correct ectropion or entropion.[5]

2. Prosthokeratoplasty

The globe may require prosthokeratoplasty if corneal grafts fail to construct the anterior segment.

3. Facial Reconstructive Surgery

The face may require reconstruction of abnormalities by use of local skin flaps and distant split-thickness skin flaps.

REFERENCES

1. **Abt, J. L.,** The pupillary responses after being struck by lightning, *JAMA*, 254, 3312, 1985.
2. **Tribble, C. G., Persing, J. A., Morgan, R. F., Kenney, J. G., and Edlich, R. F.,** Lightning injuries, *Compr. Ther.,* 11, 32, 1985.
3. **Fraunfelder, F. T.,** Electrical injury, in *Current Ocular Therapy 3,* Fraunfelder, F. T. and Roy, F. H., Eds., W. B. Saunders, Philadelphia, 1989.
4. **Krob, M. J. and Cram, A. E.,** Lightning injuries: a multisystem trauma, *J. Iowa Med. Soc.,* 73, 221, 1983.
5. **Marrone, A. C.,** Thermal eyelid burns, in *Oculoplastic, Orbital and Reconstructive Surgery,* Hornblass, A., Ed., Williams & Wilkins, Baltimore, 1988, chap. 49.
6. **Saffle, J. R., Crandall, A., and Warden, G. D.,** Cataracts: a long-term complication of electrical injury, *J. Trauma,* 25, 17, 1985.
7. **Fraunfelder, F. T. and Hanna, C.,** Electric cataracts. I. Sequential changes, unusual and prognostic findings, *Arch. Ophthalmol.,* 87, 179, 1972.
8. **Raymond, L. F.,** Specific treatment of uveitis, lightning induced: an auto-immune disease, *Ann. Allergy,* 27, 242, 1969.

VI. TREATMENT OF COCHLEOVESTIBULAR INJURY FROM LIGHTNING

LaV. Bergstrom

The patient may be unconscious and may have no heartbeat. Resuscitation of the patient using cardiopulmonary techniques and electric shock to the chest wall to restore a normal rhythm is essential in these critical cases. Cardiopulmonary resuscitation may be continued while the patient is being transported to a facility where cardioversion and antiarrhythmic drugs can be administered and the patient monitored.

Victims of lightning strike may have minor arrhythmias, bleeding, or cerebrospinal fluid (CSF) coming from the ears, and may be disoriented and uncooperative while being examined. The otologist cannot have the patient transferred to the otological clinic, but can have the operating microscope and appropriate ear instruments brought to the bedside of the patient if the otoscope does not give an adequate view. Often, there is a clot in the external ear canal which must be evacuated before a complete examination can be done. Tuning fork testing should be done at the bedside as soon as possible to get some idea of the hearing loss. Patients will often complain of roaring or high-pitched tinnitus and may find it somewhat difficult to localize to tuning forks, but this problem can be minimized by using a 512-Hz tuning fork. Vertigo also is a fairly common symptom. Sometimes, local soft tissue or bony loss and partial avulsion of the pinna may make it difficult to examine the ear canal and drum. Local tissue may be available, and the partial avulsion of the pinna should be sutured. An audiogram may need to be delayed until local tissues have healed and are no longer painful. Quite frequently, there is a tympanic membrane perforation, sometimes with the edges inverted into the middle ear. This can be manipulated into an everted position, but is best done in a few days when the patient is stable and out of the intensive care unit. A four-quadrant block with a local anesthetic of about 1.5 to 2.0-cc volume combined with 1:100,000 injectable epinephrine will usually provide adequate analgesia. Care must be taken to explain to the patient just before each needle stick is done that some pain will occur early, but that as the injection proceeds, the pain will usually decrease. The needle should be $1^1/_2$ to $1^3/_4$ in. long, 27 gauge in diameter, and disposable. Eardrum blanching due to the epinephrine may not occur in these cases, or there may be subtotal blanching. Perforation or avulsion of a portion of the tympanic membrane may occur in any area.

Charring of the ear canal is sometimes seen, and there may be bleeding between the layers of the eardrum, although this is quite rare. It is tempting to consider early exploration of the middle ear and performance of tympanoplasty. However, lightning injury of the tympanic membrane has some similarities to welding injuries of the ear in that there is marked edema, burning and charring of the external auditory canal and drum, and other inflammatory changes which suggest damage to the local vasculature. Spontaneous healing of the perforation may occur.

Other traumas to the temporal bone include permanent disruption of the facial nerve with temporary or permanent paralysis, and temporal bone fracture into the labyrinth, which might cause meningitis if pathogenic organisms in the middle ear or in a deep laceration in continuity with the fracture occur. Nearby facial burns might also be infected and spread organisms to the ear. A culture of the CSF issuing from the ear should be done as well as a culture of spinal fluid obtained by lumbar puncture. Early antibiotic coverage can be changed when the results of cultures and sensitivities are known. Middle ear ossicles may be dislocated or fractured; this can often be diagnosed using computerized axial tomography. Reconstruction using the ossicles themselves or prosthetic replacement could be done at tympanoplasty or at a second stage in 6 to 12 months after the tympanic membrane perforation is healed.

While the tympanic membrane is perforated, dry-ear precautions must be observed. When showering or shampooing, a shower cap should be used in combination with a cotton plug sealed with vaseline or other appropriate barrier. Swimming may be allowed if the patient will use earplugs and wear a tightly fitting swimming cap. Diving is precluded.

Hearing acuity often improves and tinnitus may lessen, but in a moderate hearing loss that involves more than one or two high frequencies, hearing aids may be needed, especially if both ears have significant hearing loss. If there is total bilateral deafness, a cochlear implant might be appropriate if there is no significant vestibular damage. Vestibular symptoms may be a feature of the early course of lightning injury, but because the vestibular system includes the cerebellum, spinocerebellar tracts, vision, and proprioception, substantive recovery may be anticipated as the system makes adjustments. However, if the cerebullum, vision, or proprioception are also damaged, recovery may not occur or may occur partially after a protracted time. Also, if the involvement is bilateral, recovery is unlikely. Age, arthritis, or decreased mental acuity may also impede or retard recovery. Physical therapy may be of some value to selected patients.

If there is extensive cardiac or cerebral injury, the prognosis is extremely poor.

VII. SPECIAL MANAGEMENT OF BURNS

S. P. Pegg

A. MANAGEMENT PRINCIPLES

Severe burns in lightning injury are the exception rather than the rule. This section will concentrate on treatment of burns when they do occur. The management of burns following lightning injuries is an extension of the previous resuscitation in the emergency room or intensive care unit. In treating the burn injury, other aspects of the lightning injury must take precedence. The priorities are very much the treatment of associated injuries and complications while the burn injuries are being assessed and treated with antimicrobial creams. Myocardial damage is not uncommon and may be reflected in ECG abnormalities and dysrhythmias, and this aspect must be treated as top priority, with ECG monitoring and with monitoring of the cardiac isoenzyme levels.[1] Abnormalities of cardiac rhythm may persist until the patient is discharged.[2]

In lightning injury, damage to skeletal muscle may, in rare instances, be reflected in myoglobinuria. The immediate need with this present is to protect the kidneys by adequate resuscitation and increasing the urine output. Yost and Holmes[3] stress the need to protect the kidneys by the use of osmotic diuretics and by alkalinizing the urine. The possibility of renal failure is important and needs to be monitored closely, but may occur more frequently with hypotension than with myoglobinuria. Tympanic membrane rupture[4,5] need not delay the actual treatment. However, neurological lesions may well delay surgery because of risks associated with anesthesia during this acute phase.

B. RESUSCITATION

Cardiopulmonary resuscitation, having been initiated as early as possible, should continue until there is full assessment of cerebral function, and fluid administration should be adequate. Because of the possibility of damage to muscle masses with subsequent fluid loss in these areas, the fluid requirements may be much greater than indicated by the usual formulas used in resuscitation. A standard formula regimen for fluid replacement may be used to institute fluid management, and should be instituted as and when indicated.

If there are deep burns, fluid requirements may be much greater than otherwise thought, due to severe muscle edema, and should be increased as indicated by urine output, blood pressure and pulse-rate monitoring, and by readings from the central venous pressure monitoring if this has been instituted. In the first 24 h, generally normal saline or lactated Ringer's solution is given. However, if indicated by the fall of blood pressure, do not hesitate to give colloid solution. If myoglobinuria is present, the urine output should be increased from the normal 30 to 70-ml/h requirement to at least 100 ml/h by increasing the intravenous fluids, and this should be continued until the urine is clear. For children, the usual urine output of 1 ml/kg of body weight per hour will need to be doubled until the urine is clear. Fluid administration should nevertheless be balanced against the exacerbation of cerebral edema.

C. TETANUS PROPHYLAXIS

Tetanus prophylaxis must be instituted as early as possible after the accident. This should include tetanus immunoglobulin and tetanus toxoid.

D. ANTIBIOTICS

With the risk of electric and traumatic muscle damage, there is an increased risk of bacterial gangrene, and penicillin should be used prophylactically (1-M units, intravenously, 8 hourly) with these patients, accompanied by early treatment of any burn wound and excision of any dead tissue. Other problems such as myocardial damage or neurological injury may, of course, delay taking the patient to the operating theater.

E. BURN WOUND

There may be a definite entrance and exit wound, sometimes with extensive damage, particularly near the exit wound. Rarely, there may be patchy necrosis occurring beneath unaffected skin. However, the immediate apparent problem will be treatment of the full-thickness burns at entry and exit sites. Added to this, however, are the arborizing and serpiginous patterns of dermal burn, giving a fern-like appearance as they branch away from a central area.[2,8] These fern-like superficial burns heal rapidly within a few days and do not cause problems. Other patterns include the linear burn, which is usually partial thickness. Transient erythema and burns from contact with metal apparel may also be seen. The latter may be full thickness.

1. Full-Thickness Burns

Full-thickness burns, usually small in area, are seen at entry and exit sites, and also arising from metal contact.

a. Skin Grafting

Generally, skin grafting will not be needed. The superficial fern-like burns will heal rapidly, and some full-thickness burns may be of such a nature that they also will heal rapidly,[5] e.g., very narrow burns. However, when full-thickness skin loss occurs, the skin usually should be excised and grafted as soon as practicable. This is performed under a general anesthetic or neurolept anesthetic, and skin grafts taken with an air dermatome to a thickness of 12 to 14/1000 in. applied. Whether the skin graft is meshed for this grafting procedure will, of course, depend to a large extent on the area involved, i.e., its size and whether blood is oozing from the surface. Generally, the area to be skin grafted is not too great. If there is a very deep loss in a small essential area, such as over a wrist joint, then the use of rotational flaps or even free flaps to provide good, quick cover should be considered. The area of the injury, the availability of suitable flaps, and the overall general condition of the patient will help dictate whether these will be used. The use of antimicrobial creams can allow the patient to be stabilized before the operation is necessary and will keep the bacterial count at a low enough level to allow safe, early excision and grafting.

Grafts can be kept in place by using chlorhexidine tulle over the graft and then using skin staples to attach the graft, with a nonadhesive dressing over this, held in place by bandages. Grafts are generally taken down and inspected 2 or 3 d after grafting, depending on the possibility of infection.

b. Escharotomy and Fasciotomy

Escharotomy and fasciotomy, while not usually needed, may be indicated in an affected limb where considerable edema and tenderness may indicate deep muscle damage. If equipment is readily available for compartmental pressure measurements, this may be used. A diagnosis of a compartment syndrome is rare in pure lightning injury, and must be entertained cautiously. Escharotomy and fasciotomy may only then be appropriate, and if performed, are then regarded as burn wounds themselves. They are covered with antiseptic tulle and packed with antimicrobial cream such as silver sulfadiazine cream with antiseptic. At a later stage, it may be possible to close these incisions, or they can be skin grafted in any subsequent grafting procedure.

Amputations, like fasciotomies, are not common in lightning injury, but if a limb is dead, then amputation will be necessary. The diagnosis is again approached with caution. An arteriogram and a radioactive technetium scan may help determine the level of amputation. Amputations can be delayed for a few days, and the timing may depend on the overall condition of the patient, particularly in relation to the myocardial and neurological problems.

2. Partial-Thickness Burns

Linear burns are mostly partial thickness in severity. The partial-thickness burn wound should be carefully cleaned with aqueous chlorhexidine solution or other suitable antimicrobial solutions. Loose dead tissue should be excised and a topical antimicrobial cream applied such as Silvazine® (Smith & Nephew), which contains silver sulfadiazine cream (1% w/w) with chlorhexidine digluconate (0.2% w/w). Other antimicrobial creams are available and could be used. Affected limbs should be elevated to approximately 15° above the horizontal to help limit possible edema, and splints may be required at this stage to help prevent deformities from subsequently developing. Contractures can readily develop not only from any serious burn scars, but also as a result of rare ischemic necrosis of damaged muscles.

F. REHABILITATION

Once the areas have been skin grafted and the skin can accept a pressure garment, the latter should be commenced as indicated to help prevent hypertrophic scars; it will be necessary to wear the garment until the scar is mature, which may be 9 to 12 months. Wearing splints at night may be necessary for some time to prevent contractures, but this should be stopped as soon as possible to allow return to as near normal activities as can be achieved. Vigorous physiotherapy for affected limbs may be required from the time of injury until full rehabilitation occurs, and will be dictated by the area of injury. Psychological support, not only for burn injuries, will be necessary for these patients if they are to achieve full rehabilitation. With the traumatic nature of the injury, and with possible deafness from tympanic rupture as well as surgery being required, psychological support is a most important element in the total treatment of these patients. Burn and other support groups can be very helpful.

G. SUMMARY

All efforts should be made to ensure the early cardiopulmonary resuscitation of these patients, with vigorous, adequate fluid resuscitation and investigation of their many problems. The aim of treatment is to allow speedy rehabilitation.

REFERENCES

1. **Jackson, S. H. D. and Parry, J.,** Lightning and the heart, *Br. Heart J.,* 43, 454, 1980.
2. **Amy, B. W., McManus, W. F., Goodwin, C. W., and Pruitt, B.,** Lightning injury with survival in a few patients, *JAMA,* 253, 243, 1985.
3. **Yost, J. W. and Holmes, F. F.,** Myoglobinuria following lightning stroke, *JAMA,* 228, 1147, 1974.
4. **Wright, J. W. and Silk, K. L.,** Acoustic and vestibular defects in lightning survivors, *Laryngoscope,* 84, 1378, 1974.
5. **Agnew, J.,** Lightning injury, *Proc. Div. Surg. R. Brisbane Hosp.,* 2, 61, 1986.
6. **Baxter, C. R.,** Fluid volume and electrolyte changes in the early postburn period, *Clin. Plast. Surg.,* 1, 693, 1974.
7. **Robson, M. C.,** Discussion — electrical injury mechanisms, *Plast. Reconstr. Surg.,* 80, 5, 680, 1987.
8. **ten Duis, H. J., Klase, H. J., and Nijsten, M. W. N.,** Superficial lightning injuries — their 'fractal' shape and origin, *Burns,* 13, 2, 141, 1987.

VIII. PSYCHOLOGICAL MANAGEMENT OF LIGHTNING VICTIMS

S. J. Dollinger

A. INTRODUCTION

Natural disasters have been conceptualized by Lifton and Olson[8] as involving five dimensions: (1) the suddenness or unpredictability of the disaster, (2) relationship of the disaster to irresponsibility or callousness of individuals or groups of people (the question of human agency), (3) whether there is a continuing relationship to the disaster (e.g., economic consequences in the community), (4) the isolation of the community, and (5) the totality of the disaster. Unless there are extraordinary circumstances, lightning incidents will tend to fall at the least traumatic end of these dimensions, particularly as compared with such events as earthquakes. Tornados and floods will tend to hold an intermediate position on the disaster continuum. Consequently, lightning strike trauma will be somewhat less likely to lead to major psychological problems. But like all traumatic events, it will often lead to at least transient symptoms of anxiety, such as disturbed sleep, somatic complaints, specific fears, or generalized worries, and has the potential for causing more lasting emotional difficulties.

Among the five disaster dimensions, unpredictability will often play a part in lightning incidents, making them more traumatic. But the second dimension will usually be most important: a lightning injury will be psychologically more traumatic to the extent that human agency can be thought to have been involved. In the incident with which this writer is most familiar, the lightning strike occurred during a children's soccer game which had been postponed during a thunderstorm. The incident followed a decision by coaches and referees to resume the game after the rain had ceased and the overhead sky had cleared. When the lightning struck, all of the players and those on the sidelines were knocked to the ground and 3 of the 38 players required hospitalization; one child never regained consciousness and died 1 week later. Thus, the circumstances of the incident were sufficiently ambiguous and the outcome sufficiently severe to cause some people to second guess the decision to resume. In this case, the second guessing primarily took the form of self-blame by those who helped make the decision. Other adults who were present typically felt that the decision made sense at the time, especially after having "waited out" the storm. Nevertheless, the human agency element played a clear role.

B. DIAGNOSIS AND TREATMENT

All traumatic events have the potential to cause transient distress. This distress in its mildest forms will include such problems as nightmares, insomnia, vague aches and pains (e.g., in the stomach or head), and sadness or crying associated with recurrent thoughts about the incident. Such problems were common in the sample studied by the author[3] and are consistent with the report of another research team.[9] If the frequency and intensity of these symptoms becomes distressing to the victim or his/her family and persist for at least 1 month, they could constitute reasonable grounds for considering a diagnosis of post-traumatic stress disorder (PTSD) as described in the latest edition of the American Psychiatric Association's Diagnostic and Statistical Manual (DSM-III-R).[1] (PTSD with delayed onset would be considered if symptoms began 6 months after the trauma.) Aside from the presence of a trauma and the 1-month duration, three categories of phenomena are considered. First, the traumatic event is persistently reexperienced. This could involve flashback episodes (sudden feeling that the event is recurring), intrusive recollections about it, distressing dreams, or distress at the symbolic exposure to the event, including anniversaries of the trauma. Second, there is persistent avoidance of stimuli associated with the trauma. (Three of seven possible referents are considered; the reader is referred to DSM-III-R for specific examples of this category.) And finally, the diagnosis requires at least two of six possible symptoms, where these symptoms were not present prior to the traumatic event: (1) insomnia, (2) irritability/angry outbursts, (3) difficulty concentrating, (4) hypervigilance, (5) exaggerated startle response, and (6) physiological reactivity to events that resemble or symbolize the trauma. Depending upon the circumstances and the condition of the individual patient, treatment might consist of some combination of individual, group, or family therapy and medication.

If the victim's response does not qualify for the diagnosis because of lesser duration or severity, adjustment disorder would be diagnosed.[1] Among the sample of youngsters seen by this writer, about 80% (30/38) could be thought to have shown some degree of upset by the lightning incident, but even the most upset group (comprising about 20%) would more clearly fall into the DSM-III-R adjustment disorder than the PTSD diagnostic category. Aside from the boy who died, the two who were hospitalized had quite different emotional reactions to it, although neither had a memory for the incident.[3,7] One had a very bland reaction (and from all indications and reports, this was typical of his style before the incident). The other developed depression of sufficient severity to warrant a 1-month hospitalization. This was thought by physicians to be due to physiological rather than psychological factors, and this child's response would not qualify for PTSD. Others among the most upset group had intense symptoms of several months' duration involving phobias about weather, anxiety upon separation from parents, and, in one case, nocturnal enuresis (in a 12-year-old). With two exceptions, the problems seen in this sample resolved without any psychological intervention. One child was seen for several counseling sessions by his family physician. Another child had developed a fear of sleeping alone during thunderstorms and his mother requested referral 6 months after the incident. (Such a problem might be thought of as a delayed effect of trauma or as a reflection of a family interaction difficulty) It should be noted, however, that therapeutic benefits might have obtained from participation in the research interview. Many families seemed to use the interview to express feelings about and try to come to grips emotionally with the tragedy; and these families seemed appreciative of the opportunity to tell their stories.

Although diagnosable problems resolved, it is worth noting that the children's sense of general vulnerability to life events may have been affected. For example, natural disasters can increase fears that remain at a subclinical level or influence one's sense of the likelihood of future negative events. Those in the lightning sample completed a fear survey shortly after their interviews (1 to 2 months post-disaster) and their answers were compared to nonvictims of comparable age, sex, and socioeconomic status.[5] The lightning victims had significantly greater fears of storms, animals, noisy events, supernatural phenomena (ghosts), and enclosed spaces, plus greater sleep-related fears, bodily penetration anxiety, and fears of death or dying. An 8-year follow-up was conducted by one of the writer's students.[6] This research found that, as they were about to graduate from high school, these young people still had a greater sense that lightning might "kill someone like me"— their subjective probability of vulnerability seems to be a lasting one.

Should a lightning victim seek counseling, a number of treatment options can be considered. In the case of virtually all victims of traumatic stress, the opportunity to talk about their memories and feelings concerning the incident is essential. The listener (counselor) should convey understanding, respect, and a wish to be of help.[11] The general notion of emotional catharsis for traumatic events is commonly endorsed by therapists of various orientations, and it has research support to back it up.[10] Beyond such "nonspecific" treatment, problem-solving therapy might be of use to effect some mitigation of symptoms such as fears, nightmares, or flashback experiences. This therapy might include the assistance of the victim's family members in changing the environment or its reinforcement contingencies to encourage other behaviors. Or the focus could be on desensitizing the victim to stimuli associated with the lightning strike that continue to evoke fear. Quite possibly, systematic desensitization could be helpful in this regard, although the preliminary relaxation training alone would be sufficient in some cases.

C. CONCLUDING REMARKS

Appreciating the psychology of being a lightning victim requires a recognition of the "human meanings" of traumatic events.[8] Because people are not passive recipients of life events, the victims of tragic and traumatic happenings will be experiencing intense and distressing emotions in part because of how they construe what happened and why. In particular, there is concern with whether blame can or should be assigned.[2,4,12] A corollary to the point about human meanings is that the psychological victims of a lightning strike incident will often include the family members of those directly hit and any persons who have witnessed the incident. Thus, the psychology of lightning disaster involves some understanding of people's grief and response to death.

REFERENCES

1. **American Psychiatric Association,** *Diagnostic and Statistical Manual of Mental Disorders,* 3rd ed., revised (DSM-III-R), Washington, D.C., 1987.
2. **Bulman, R. J. and Wortman, C. B.,** Attributions of blame and coping in the "real world": severe accident victims react to their lot, *J. Pers. Soc. Psychol.,* 35, 351, 1977.
3. **Dollinger, S. J.,** Lightning-strike disaster among children, *Br. J. Med. Psychol.,* 58, 375, 1985.
4. **Dollinger, S. J.,** The need for meaning following disaster: attributions and emotional upset, *Pers. Soc. Psychol. Bull.,* 12, 300, 1986.
5. **Dollinger, S. J., O'Donnell, J. P., and Staley, A. A.,** Lightning-strike disaster: effects on children's fears and worries, *J. Consult. Clin. Psychol.,* 52, 1028, 1984.
6. **Greening, L.,** Adolescent's Perceptions of Fatal Risks: An Evaluation of the Availability Heuristic, Ph.D. thesis, Southern Illinois University, Carbondale, 1988.
7. **Kotagal, S., Rawlings, C. A., Chen, S., Burris, G., and Nouri, S.,** Neurologic, psychiatric, and cardiovascular complications in children struck by lightning, *Pediatrics,* 70, 190, 1982.
8. **Lifton, R. J. and Olson, E.,** The human meaning of total disaster, *Psychiatry,* 39, 1, 1976.
9. **Myers, G. J., Colgan, M. T., and VanDyke, D. H.,** Lightning-strike disaster among children, *JAMA,* 238, 1045, 1977.
10. **Pennebaker, J. W. and Beall, S. K.,** Confronting a traumatic event: toward an understanding of inhibition and diseases, *J. Abnorm. Psychol.,* 95, 274, 1986.
11. **Reisman, J. M.,** *Toward the Integration of Psychotherapy,* John Wiley & Sons, New York, 1971.
12. **Taylor, S. E.,** Adjustment to threatening events: a theory of cognitive adaptation, *Am. Psychol.,* 38, 1161, 1983.

Chapter 8

LIGHTNING INJURIES — FOLLOW-UP AND PROGNOSIS

Mary Ann Cooper

TABLE OF CONTENTS

I. GENERAL PROGNOSIS

The minimally injured lightning victim in general needs only a good physical examination, observation, either in the hospital or by a responsible family member if the injuries are minor enough, and referral for any conditions that may need further evaluation, such as tympanic membrane rupture.

The more moderately injured patient may need hospitalization for a few days while the injuries are evaluated, monitored, and a rehabilitation plan is designed, if necessary.

The most severely injured victims have a variable prognosis. Those who respond rapidly to resuscitation or who are young and otherwise healthy may do quite well, although with varying levels of sequelae. Patients who do not respond as well generally have a poor prognosis and, of those who survive hospitalization, many have severe permanent sequelae, including paresis, seizures, and vegetative states.

II. SPECIFIC FOLLOW-UP

A. CARDIAC

Most patients who have had electrocardiographic changes (specifically, ST changes) on initial presentation will have these clear within 6 months or less. Seldom will these be clinically significant after the patient has survived the first few days without arrhythmias. It is extremely rare for patients to have continuing problems with congestive heart failure or other cardiac problems unless they have had underlying cardiac disease.

B. NEUROLOGIC

Some patients may complain of continuing pain and weakness in an extremity injured by the lightning stroke. They may also complain of weakness, but it is unclear if this is primary or is secondary to pain on use of the extremity. These symptoms are probably due to neuropathy because of peripheral nerve ischemia or damage at the time of the stroke, but, while it is a common complaint, few neurologists or physicians have been interested enough to evaluate it completely to date. Nonsteroidal, antiinflammatory drugs are generally used for this with limited success. Electromyography and other testing may be appropriate in order to define the extent of disability and to plan rehabilitation. Sometimes this condition clears with time, sometimes it is permanent, and to date there is nothing in the literature that gives a guide to predicting the prognosis.

Occasionally, the patient who showed keraunoparalysis on initial presentation will have permanent paresis and will need to have physical therapy to regain maximal function.

Lightning victims who have seizures as a result of some correctable problem such as hypoxia due to a temporarily obstructed airway will not be bothered with them afterwards. However, patients who have seizures because of brain damage have the same prognosis as any patient with a similar traumatic or hypoxic lesion and should be treated with this in mind.

C. PSYCHIATRIC AND PSYCHOLOGICAL

Many, if not all, lightning victims have some degree of psychiatric symptomatology as a result of their experience. However, not all require psychiatric care. Many of the changes have to do with increased awareness of weather conditions and fear of storms. Other patients, however, will have more severe symptoms that may require referral for testing and therapy. These include sleep disturbances, changes in mental ability and personality, storm phobias, and irritability.

D. OPHTHALMIC

Changes in vision need to be evaluated by an ophthalmologist. Cataracts may occur, but so may a whole host of injuries, as noted in Chapters 5 and 6, which can be treated in the standard way and have a prognosis that is similar to any other traumatic cause of the same lesion.

E. OTOLOGIC

As discussed, tympanic membrane rupture, ossicular disruption, and cochlear disturbances are fairly common with lightning injuries. Those that require operative intervention are usually delayed until the edema and inflammation of the original injury have time to resolve. Until that time, they are treated conservatively and supportively. Evaluation of hearing with otologic testing may be indicated.

F. MUSCULOSKELETAL

These are treated in the usual fashion and have the same prognosis as other traumatic lesions to the musculoskeletal system.

G. BURNS

These are generally superficial and require little care. In the rare event of deep burns, they should be treated as any other electrical burn, depending on their size and extent, and may require referral to a burn center.

H. RENAL

It is uncommon to have injuries to the renal system. When they do occur, they are usually secondary to either hypotension as a result of cardiac arrest and low perfusional states or, rarely, to myoglobinuric renal failure.

I. GASTROINTESTINAL

GI symptomatology has usually cleared by the time the patient is discharged from the hospital. Otherwise, it is treated in the standard fashion as indicated by the pathology.

Chapter 9

PROTECTION FROM LIGHTNING

David Mackerras

TABLE OF CONTENTS

I. INTRODUCTION

General information on the occurrence and physical nature of lightning has been given by Golde[1] and Uman,[2] and the application of the information to lightning protection has been described by Golde.[3] This chapter sets out to show that knowledge of the processes in the lightning discharge to ground, in particular the *first leader stroke* and *first return stroke,* permit a rational approach to the protection of persons and buildings against injury or damage by lightning.

While the protection of persons and buildings are traditionally considered separately, there is some justification in considering these matters together, as the same principles are involved and persons inside buildings can be at risk. Hence, an adequate understanding of the nature of the risk is best attained by considering the two aspects together.

II. PHYSICAL BASIS FOR LIGHTNING PROTECTION

To understand the physical basis for lightning protection, we need to review certain aspects of the lightning discharge, based on the description given in Chapter 2. The *first leader stroke* of a *ground flash* progresses in a predominantly downward direction, covering the distance from the negative charge center to a point near ground typically in about 20 ms. Objects on the earth's surface appear to have little or no influence on the path of the leader until it is within about 200 m of the earth. From that height downward, salient objects on the earth's surface may influence the downward path by affecting the electric field between the advancing tip of the leader and earth. The electric charge distributed along the leader channel creates a strong electric field at the surface of the earth. This field will be enhanced at the upper and outer parts of objects protruding from the surface of the earth, such as buildings, towers, overhead power or communications conductors, or persons in the open. At some of these exposed points, electrical discharges in the form of upward streamers will be initiated by the electric field. These streamers will grow in the general direction of the tip of the leader stroke. One of these streamers, or occasionally two or more streamers, will succeed in reaching the downcoming leader tip. At this point, the currents in the streamers will rise from a value of a few tens or hundreds of amperes to the peak value of the lightning current in the range of a few thousand to about 100,000 A.

A *lightning strike attachment point* is the position from which the successful streamer originates, i.e., the streamer that succeeds in reaching the downcoming leader. The full lightning current flows at this attachment point. If more than one streamer succeeds in reaching the downcoming leader, the current will be shared between the paths thus established. Assuming for simplicity that there is only one successful streamer and attachment point, one can see that the position of the bottom portion of the lightning channel has been determined by the path of the successful upward streamer, and hence by the object from which the streamer originated. The object being struck by lightning therefore plays an active role in determining the position in space of the lower portion of the lightning channel. An elevated earthed object will divert to itself any lightning that would otherwise have struck the ground in the absence of the object. An elevated earthed object thus establishes in its vicinity a *zone of protection,* i.e., a volume of space into which a lightning channel does not penetrate. For objects of moderate height (less than about 15 m), the zone of protection has an approximately conical form, with the apex at the tip of the elevated earthed object. For larger objects, the *rolling sphere method* of determining the zone of protection is applicable. This method is explained in Section X.

Thus, the physical basis for *interception lightning protection* is to position earthed conductors at points that will control the path of the bottom end of the lightning discharge. These conducting parts may already exist in the situation requiring protection, or they may have to be deliberately placed so as to provide launching points for streamers. The remainder of the task in interception lightning protection is to provide conducting paths to earth for the lightning current. The task of providing interception lightning protection may be considered to be successfully accomplished if there is a high probability that any lightning flash to the situation being protected will terminate on one of the earthed conductors deliberately provided, or already existing, and that the lightning current will flow harmlessly to earth through downconductors and earth electrodes. Various national standards on lightning protection[4-7] give detailed requirements for the design, installation, and maintenance of lightning protection systems.

III. MECHANISMS FOR THE INTERCEPTION OF PART OR ALL OF THE LIGHTNING CURRENT BY A PERSON

A. INTERCEPTION BY A PERSON OF MOST OR ALL OF A LIGHTNING DISCHARGE CURRENT

This situation exists where the person becomes the primary lightning strike attachment point, usually on the upper portion of the body, and will be associated with situations where persons are in the open, on foot, or on an unprotected vehicle. The person will thus be subjected to the full lightning current, or a substantial fraction of it where there are two or more channels to ground. The injuries to be expected are detailed in Chapter 5.

The current delivered at the stroke attachment point will divide between paths inside the body and over the surface of the body, as explained in Chapters 3 and 6. The presence of films of sweat on the skin, and the presence of damp and somewhat conductive clothing in the path of the current favor a superficial path. It is intuitively plausible that injuries will be lessened as a greater fraction of the current flows in superficial paths.

B. INTERCEPTION BY A PERSON OF A RELATIVELY SMALL PORTION OF THE LIGHTNING DISCHARGE CURRENT

Several situations exist where the person is subjected to only a fraction of the total lightning current. Where there is a conducting path carrying most of the lightning current and the person's position is such that a fraction of the current passes through the body, the effects will depend on the magnitude and characteristics of the total current, the fraction that is diverted through the body, and the path through the body. Direct contact with the main current path is not a necessary condition, as a short discharge through air (side flash) may complete the path for the current.

A "touch potential" effect will exist where the person's hand touches one part of the main lightning current path, and the feet complete the path through the body. The diverted current will then pass through the trunk of the body.

A "step potential" effect will exist where the lightning current path is through the ground, away from the strike attachment point, and the person's feet contact points on the ground at different potentials. As the current path is then up one leg and down the other, there is less danger to abdominal or thoracic organs than with touch potential. However, with quadruped animals, step potential can be lethal.

When a person is swimming or wading and lightning strikes the water nearby, current flows through the water away from the strike point. Part of the lightning current will then flow through the body, with a path that depends on the position of the body in the water in relation to the strike point. Conditions are likely to favor a substantial current flow through the body, rather than over the surface of the body, and this situation is generally considered very dangerous.

IV. OTHER MECHANISMS FOR PRODUCING CURRENT FLOW IN THE BODY

A. FORMATION OF AN UNSUCCESSFUL STREAMER FROM A PERSON'S HEAD

In a situation where there is a lightning strike near a person in an open field, an unsuccessful upward streamer may arise from the person's head during the last stage of the downward progression of the first leader stroke. An unsuccessful upward streamer of this type would cause a current flow of the order of 10 to 100 A, lasting a few tens or hundreds of microseconds, through the trunk and head of the person. One can only speculate as to the effect this would have on the person. Some such mechanisms may help to explain the following observation.

At Marchant Park, in the northern part of Brisbane, Australia, a lightning flash from a thundercloud about 3 km away struck and killed one of the players at a cricket match. A person serving at a nearby kiosk observed this event and reported that all the other players in the vicinity of the stricken person collapsed slowly and lay stunned on the ground for a period, then gradually got back on their feet. It is likely that each player so affected had an unsuccessful upward streamer from their head, and each suffered temporary unconsciousness, but no permanent ill effect, from this. Of course, this is merely speculation, and an alternative mechanism could be that the large values of rate of change of magnetic field, electric field, or both induced a current in the brain that had the effect of causing temporary unconsciousness.

B.   NONELECTRICAL EFFECTS OF LIGHTNING ON PERSONS

Nonelectrical effects of lightning include acoustic, mechanical, thermal, and optical radiation effects. The acoustic radiation close to a return stroke channel has been described in Chapter 2. Mechanical effects can result from the sudden conversion of moisture into high-pressure steam, resulting in the disruption of wood or other materials. Injury to persons may then result from dislodged material traveling at high speed away from the lightning current path. Thus, persons have been injured by fragments of a tree trunk ejected by lightning current. The thermal-optical radiation from a lightning channel corresponds to that of a few centimeters-diameter column of heated gas at a temperature of about 30,000 K for the first few microseconds of the return stroke, falling to about 10,000 K after a few hundred microseconds. In addition to radiation energy, direct contact between a person's skin and the end of the return stroke channel will result in heating by conduction from the heated gas in the discharge channel.

V. EFFECTS OF LIGHTNING CURRENT ON PARTS OF STRUCTURES

The principal effect of lightning current on the parts of structures is thermal, as a result of the deposition of energy, $\int i^2 R dt$, in any path having resistance R as explained in Chapter 3. If the limits of integration are the times of start and finish of the flash, and R remains constant, the energy can be expressed as

$$w = \left[\int i^2 dt \right] R$$

The quantity $\int i^2 dt$ is known as the action integral. The median value is about 5×10^3 A^{2}s, implying that about 5 kJ will be deposited in a 1-Ω resistor by the passage of a typical lightning current, while in an extremely severe flash, about 500 kJ would be deposited.[8,9] Heating effects can be calculated on this basis for a given material and the dimensions of the conducting path. A copper wire of diameter 2 mm will just be melted by the passage of a severe lightning flash current. Thus, the requirement in AS1768[5] for a 35-mm cross-sectional area for a conductor installed to carry the full lightning current is quite conservative, and is based mainly on a requirement for mechanical durability and limiting the temperature rise to safe values.

Most metal parts of buildings are able to carry lightning currents without any harmful effect, the only exception being that where the lightning strike attaches to a thin metal surface, a hole may be melted. For example, a severe lightning current, transferring 70 C of charge, would melt a hole about 100 mm^2 in area in a sheet of galvanized iron 0.38 mm^2 thick.[3] In contrast, lightning currents can produce very harmful effects in more resistive materials, producing localized heating along the current path. Where moisture is present, high-pressure steam will be generated, with disruptive effects on the material. This is believed to be the mechanism whereby pieces of concrete or stonework are dislodged by lightning. In dry materials, or where the lightning current passes through air as an arc, high temperatures are generated that may initiate a fire or an explosion. The passage of lightning current through highly resistive materials in a building will be associated with large potential differences between adjacent parts of the building, with consequent hazard to occupants and electrical equipment, as well as the fabric of the building.

Any conductor carrying lightning current will be subjected to an electromagnetic force $F = Bli$ (newton), where l is the length of the conductor (meter), i is the current (ampere), and B is the component of the magnetic field (tesla) at right angles to the conductor. The force is at right angles to both the conductor and B. The magnetic field will be generated by the complete lightning current flow pattern in the situation under consideration. In some situations, these forces need to be considered, but it is generally found that they do not create a problem in lightning protection systems. For example, normal methods of fastening air termination conductors and downconductors to a building are sufficient to secure the conductors against electromagnetic forces.

There is always a change in the electrical potential of a structure with respect to remote earth potential when the structure is struck by lightning. As lightning usually injects negative charge into the structure (i.e., the current delivered to the structure is of negative polarity), the change in potential is usually in the negative direction with respect to remote earth. Despite this, the change is conventionally referred to as a rise in potential, ignoring the negative polarity, as will be adopted here, and potentials are understood to be relative to remote earth potential. The relation between the potential developed across an object carrying current, and the current, has been explained in Chapter 3. When applied to lightning current flowing through a structure to earth, the following effects occur.

A. RESISTIVE EFFECTS

If the structure has significant resistance in the path of the current, or if there is resistance between the structure and remote earth (earth resistance), then a potential rise $V_R = iR$ will occur, where i is the instantaneous value of lightning current (A) and R is the sum of resistances in the path of the current (Ω). For example, if $i = 80$ kA, the peak current in a moderately severe lightning flash,[10] and $R = 10\,\Omega$, a value used as an upper limit of allowed earth resistance for some classes of structure, then

$$V_R = iR = 80kA \times 10\Omega = 800kV$$

This type of potential rise is not affected by mutual coupling effects, so is the the potential difference that would occur between the structure and an isolated conductor entering the structure with its remote end at remote earth potential. Most of this resistive potential rise exists between the structure as a whole and remote earth in a structure that has adequate lightning protection.

B. INDUCTIVE EFFECTS

Any structure with appreciable vertical height will have *inductance, L (henry),* between the points at which the lightning current enters and leaves the structure, usually the top and bottom of the structure. Consequently, there will be potential V_L between these points given by

$$V_L = Ldi / dt$$

where di/dt is the instantaneous rate of change of current with respect to time (A/s). The effect is most likely to become important in a structure a few tens of meters in height. If the structure can be approximated as a vertical conducting cylindrical shell of radius r, situated on a horizontal conducting plane, the order of magnitude of the inductance per unit length will be

$$L_1 = 2\times10^{-7}\ln(2\,h\,/\,r)$$

in henry per meter, where h is the height of the portion of the building under consideration. A moderately severe lightning flash has a maximum di/dt value of about 100 GA/s.[10] If this lightning flash strikes a structure that can be approximated as a cylinder 40 m high (h) and 10 m radius (r), then the order of magnitude of the inductance per unit length halfway up the building is 3×10^{-7} H/m, and the order of magnitude of the voltage across a 1-m section of the building is $V = L_1 di/dt = 3\times10^{-7}\times10^{11} = 3\times10^4$ V. The complete potential difference from the top to the bottom of the building would be obtained by summing all contributions of this sort.

Thus, large potential differences exist across the structure during the short time for which di/dt is large, this time usually being between about 1 and 10 µs. However, magnetic and electric coupling between the structure and conductors inside it tend to maintain approximate local equipotential conditions.

C. TRANSMISSION LINE EFFECTS

For very tall structures, where the time for an electromagnetic wave to travel from the top to the bottom of the structure and back becomes comparable with the rise time of the lightning current, the structure should be modeled as a *transmission line* with *characteristic impedance* Z_o rather than as a simple inductance. The value of Z_o for a tall building is of the order of 100 Ω. The potential across the structure then becomes $V_T = iZ_o$. For example, if i = 80 kA and Z_o = 100 Ω, then $V_T = 8$ MV.

A large voltage such as the above only exists during the short-duration front of the current waveshape. The first voltage excursion may be followed by a damped train of voltage oscillations.

VI. EFFECTS OF LIGHTNING ON ELECTRICAL EQUIPMENT

Lightning can affect electrical equipment in ways that vary from momentary interference with normal operation, without any permanent effect, to total destruction of the item of equipment. The severity of the effect depends on the fraction of the lightning current entering the equipment and the ability of the equipment to withstand currents and voltages beyond normal operating values. Interference and damage can also occur to equipment by induced effects. The sudden changes of electric and magnetic fields associated with the charge movements in a lightning discharge can induce currents and voltages in exposed conductors connected to equipment, such as data lines connected to computers. A considerable body of knowledge and engineering experience has been built up concerning the protection of electric power systems, communication systems, and information processing systems against the damaging effect of lightning. So the techniques for protection are known and available,[11] although not always applied until after damage has been sustained, especially in the case of computer systems. A special case of the above is where equipment is installed in a building and lightning strikes the building. In this situation, there may be no path for any lightning current to enter the equipment, and the building may shield the equipment from electric and magnetic fields. The remaining mechanism for damage is through potential differences being applied to the equipment as a result of the potential rise of the building. These potential differences can occur between data or communication lines that have a connection to remote earth, and the equipment, whose potential will rise with the building. Similar effects can occur through the power supply lines to the equipment.

VII. PROTECTION OF PERSONS AGAINST INJURY BY LIGHTNING

The basic principle of protection of persons against lightning injury is to reduce or prevent the risk of any portion of the lightning current passing through the person. The practical application of this principle usually takes the form of defining high-risk and low-risk situations, with a recommendation that persons move quickly to a low-risk situation if caught in a high-risk situation when nearby lightning is occurring or may soon occur.

The hazard presented by a thundercloud is directly related to its ability to produce ground flashes, and this is highly variable. However, most people will have no way of knowing the degree of hazard, and should regard any thundercloud as potentially dangerous. As there are documented cases of lightning striking points on the ground up to a few kilometers away from the thundercloud, the presence of a thundercloud in the vicinity must be regarded as presenting some hazard. If ground flashes can be seen, and there is less than 15 s between flash and thunder (5-km distance), then immediate action to move to a safer position should be taken.

A. RELATIVELY LOW-RISK SITUATIONS

Any situation in which there is a substantial conducting path over and around the person, capable of intercepting the lightning discharge and conveying the current to ground without involving the person, is a relatively low-risk situation. Examples are buildings with adequate interception lightning protection, vehicles with metal parts over and around the person, and under substantial metallic structures with connections to ground, with the proviso that direct contact with the metallic structure should be avoided. A position in the open, but within the protected zone of an earthed structure, is also a low-risk situation, but not as low as inside a substantial building (see Sections II and X for an explanation of protected zones).

B. RELATIVELY HIGH-RISK SITUATIONS

Any situation in which there is a possibility that part of a person will become the lightning strike attachment point, or that a significant fraction of the lightning current will pass through the person's body, is a high-risk situation. Examples are as follows.

A position in an open field without nearby trees or other elevated objects, so that the person's head or arms become a launching point for the upward streamer, is a high-risk situation. The person, in effect, protects a surrounding area of the ground from being struck by diverting the lightning channel to himself, and receives the full lightning current through the body.

A position where the person is in contact with an object struck by lightning in such a way that a potential difference is applied to the person's body, usually between the hands and feet, is subjected to "touch potential" and is at risk to an extent that depends on the fraction of the lightning current that diverts through the body.

A position where a person's feet are subjected to a potential difference as a result of current flow through the ground away from a lightning flash is said to experience "step potential" and is at risk to an extent that depends on the position of the feet in relation to the current flow pattern in the ground. This, in turn, controls the magnitude of current through the lower parts of the body.

If a person is wading or swimming in water and lightning strikes near the person, then part of the lightning current flowing through the water will pass through the person's body. Conditions are favorable for having a relatively high fraction of the total current pass through the body.

If a person is touching an extended metal object, such as a wire fence, that is struck by lightning, then the current may travel long distances from the point of strike, and a portion of the current then flows through the person's body to ground.

A position in a small boat without metalwork overhead, and away from other, taller objects, is subject to a hazard similar to that of a person in an open field. If the boat does have metalwork overhead, such as a metal mast or metallic stays, then temporary action should be taken to make an electrical (metallic) connection of some sort from the lower end of the stays to water. For example, a length of metal chain or wire attached to a stay and with its free end in the water will provide a path to water for the lightning current. Without some such "earthing" arrangement, the occupants of the boat would be at some risk of intercepting part of the lightning current. Naturally, contact with the metal stays or metal mast should be avoided if there is a danger of close lightning. The above refers to boats with hulls made of insulating material such as fiberglass. Boats with metal hulls, of course, provide a very adequate path for the lightning current to reach the water. A boat with a metal hull and metal stays would have inherent interception lightning protection. Boats with insulating hulls can be provided with a permanent metal object, such as a keep strip, in contact with water that can be connected to the stays or metal mast. However, care must be taken that this does not result in corrosive effects on any metalwork in contact with water.

VIII. RECOMMENDED ACTIONS FOR PERSONS CAUGHT IN A HIGH-RISK SITUATION IN A THUNDERSTORM

The following recommendations are based in part on those in AS1768.[5] Persons caught in a completely open field should crouch down or squat, so as to be as low as possible, while avoiding ground currents as far as possible by contacting the ground over the smallest possible area. A sheet of insulating material, such as a plastic sheet placed on the ground where the person is sitting or crouching, will provide some protection from ground currents. If a gully or ditch is nearby, the person should get to the lowest point in it. If an isolated tree can be reached, a position several meters away from the trunk will be safer than completely in the open or right next to the trunk. A position just beyond the spread of the foliage is sometimes recommended. The tree will provide a zone of protection for the person, but there will still be some danger from flying timber if the tree is shattered, and some danger from ground currents, so the person should crouch down or sit on a sheet of plastic, if available.

If possible, the person should move quickly to a substantial building or a metal-bodied vehicle with metal overhead and around, such as a sedan car. The fact that the car has rubber tires does not prevent it from providing a high degree of protection, provided the occupants are completely inside the car and not touching the external metalwork.

Small buildings or sheds offer uncertain protection, as they often have metal roofs with no conducting path to ground. Fabric tents with supports made of electrically insulating materials similarly do not provide protection against lightning for the occupants.

Persons wading or swimming should immediately leave the water and seek a low-risk position as described above. Persons in small, open boats should seek the protection offered by a tall object such as a bridge or jetty. It is generally safer to stay in the boat, avoiding contact with the water, rather than getting into the water, for example, to pull the boat ashore.

IX. ENGINEERING ACTIONS TO REDUCE RISK TO PERSONS IN PUBLIC PLACES

In situations where large numbers of persons congregate, and there is some responsibility for protecting them from injury by lightning, there are several engineering actions that may be appropriate. Interception lightning protection may be possible for the area in question by using the zones of protection provided by tall earthed structures in the area. The effectiveness of the protection may be enhanced by using earthed overhead wires strung between existing structures or additional posts provided for the purpose. Touch-potential dangers can be minimized by providing insulating barriers to prevent persons touching or leaning on metalwork that may be carrying lightning current. Step potential can be controlled to some extent by correctly positioned conductors underground, connected to the object that may carry lightning current. Engineering actions are also applicable to situations inside buildings where the risk arises as a result of potential differences between equipment at local building potential and conductors connected to remote earth. The most commonly occurring form of this problem is the telephone, where the user of the telephone is subjected to the potential difference between the hand piece, at remote earth potential, and the surroundings, which are momentarily raised in potential by a lightning strike to the building or to power lines connected to the building. A similar situation is possible with computer users, where a data line brings in a remotely earthed conductor, while the computer or connected equipment rises in potential as a result of a lightning strike, as described above for the telephone user. In these situations, appropriately selected and positioned overvoltage protection can provide the necessary protection for persons as well as equipment.

X. PROTECTION OF STRUCTURES AGAINST DAMAGE BY LIGHTNING

The various modes of damage to structures by lightning have been outlined in Section V. The purpose of this section is to describe the main features of lightning protection for structures, with emphasis on ordinary buildings. Full details of the lightning protection required in various situations is given in national codes of lightning protection.[4-7] Interception lightning protection for a building consists of three essential parts: (1) an air termination network to intercept the lightning discharge, (2) a system of downconductors to convey the lightning current toward earth, and (3) a set of earth electrodes to deliver the current into the general mass of the earth.

Present knowledge of the sequence of events in the downward progress of the first leader, and the formation of upward streamers to complete the lightning channel to earth, has led to various methods of predicting lightning strike attachment points and the extent of the zones protected by an elevated earthed conductor by virtue of the fact that the conductor diverts to itself the lightning channel that would otherwise reach into the protected zone.

A. AIR TERMINATION NETWORK

An important concept in relation to the positioning of conductors of an air termination network is the striking distance of lightning.[3] This is the distance from the eventual strike attachment point to the tip of the downcoming leader at the moment at which it has become inevitable that the channel will bridge the gap between these two points. This distance has been estimated to be about 45 m for a lightning flash with peak current of about 10 kA,[12] although there is some controversy about this value. There is evidence that flashes with larger currents have greater striking distances and flashes with lower currents have smaller striking distances.

The *striking distance concept* can be applied in the *rolling sphere method* of determining possible strike attachment points to a building.[13] A sphere of radius equal to the assumed striking distance (usually 45 m) is imagined to be rolled across the ground and over the building. Any point touched by the sphere is a possible strike attachment point. The air termination network is designed so that the sphere can contact only air termination conductors, either existing parts of the building or conductors deliberately placed on the building as air terminations. The advantage of this method is that it is reasonably simple to apply and correctly predicts possible strike attachment points. However, being a purely geometrical method, it cannot take account of the influence of electric fields on the formation of upward streamers. As the electric field around the building will be high when the electrically charged leader stroke is close to the building, and electric field enhancement will occur at the exposed upper corners and edges of the building and at any salient object on the top, these points are the most likely upward streamer launching points. Flat surfaces near edges or corners are not likely to launch an upward streamer, although those surfaces may be touched by the rolling sphere.

For a building whose height is greater than the rolling sphere radius, the sphere will touch the sides of the building at all heights greater than the sphere radius, thus indicating a need for protection of the sides. However, strikes to the sides of a tall building are far less likely than strikes to the roof; hence, some discretion must be exercised in applying the method. One compromise is to position downconductors at the outer vertical corners, as well as at other positions, so as to serve a double purpose by also acting as air terminations for strikes to the vertical corners — the most likely position on the sides for strike attachment.[14]

B.   DOWNCONDUCTORS AND EARTHING ELECTRODES

The remainder of the lightning protection system consists of downconductors and earthing electrodes. Sufficient downconductors should be provided to ensure multiple paths around the building, giving first preference to positioning downconductors at the vertical corners. Downconductors will certainly be needed on buildings of largely nonmetallic construction. However, most large modern buildings use reinforced concrete columns, with the steel reinforcing bars forming conducting paths from the top of the building to the footings, which are usually deep in the earth. These footings provide electrical contact with the earth over a very large surface area, and are effective in dissipating lightning current to earth. Buildings without such footings will generally have to be provided with a number of metallic earth stakes, or a buried earthing conductor, to effect the transfer of lightning current into the general mass of the earth.

C.   BUILDING FEATURES THAT CONTRIBUTE TO INTERCEPTION LIGHTNING PROTECTION

As noted above, reinforced concrete columns and deep footings with reinforcing provide two important components of interception lightning protection for modern reinforced concrete buildings. Where the building also has a metal roof and a parapet covered with metal, or with a metal handrail, then a large portion of the air termination network is already present. It will then be necessary only to ensure that there are multiple electrical connections between the roof metalwork and the steel in the reinforced concrete vertical columns, preferably the peripheral ones.

Smaller buildings of largely nonmetallic construction may also have some of the elements of an interception protection system. A metal roof will usually serve as the air termination electrode. Metallic gutters and metallic downpipes to points close to the ground will serve as downconductors. To complete the protective system in such a situation, it should only be necessary to provide earth stakes connected to some downpipes, or use underground metallic pipes, to effect a connection to ground. Thus, a number of types of buildings may be protected at relatively low cost by making use of existing structural features and adding sufficient conductors to complete the protection system.

D.   BUILDING FEATURES THAT DO NOT CONTRIBUTE TO LIGHTNING PROTECTION

In general, large-scale building features of nonmetallic, nonconducting materials do not contribute to interception lightning protection. For example, a building with mainly wooden construction, a nonmetallic roof, and nonmetallic downpipes will not possess any inherent lightning protection.

A lightning strike to the roof is likely to penetrate into the space below roof level, and will probably terminate on electrical wiring in the roof, with consequent damage to electrical equipment in the building, and possible fire risk. A comparatively small amount of metallic conductor, correctly placed, will afford a high degree of protection against lightning damage in the situation described above. A wire strung across the roof of the building, following the highest parts of the roof and taken down to ground at each end, with the ends connected to metallic stakes driven into the ground (or metal water pipe running underground), will be well protected against lightning damage. The guttering, if metallic, and any substantial metal objects on the roof should be connected to the conducting system. The conductor should be reasonably substantial and durable. To satisfy AS1768,[5] it should have a cross-sectional area of at least 35 mm^2, but thinner conductors would successfully carry most lightning currents. It is interesting to note that the above is essentially the form of lightning protection for buildings described by Benjamin Franklin in 1752.

XI. CONCLUSIONS CONCERNING PROTECTION OF PERSONS AND BUILDINGS AGAINST DAMAGE BY LIGHTNING

The principles underlying the protection of both persons and buildings from injury or damage by lightning are essentially the same, being based on a knowledge of the behavior of the lightning leader stroke and the upward streamers that develop from elevated objects on the earth's surface, and thus determine the position in space of the lower end of the lightning channel to ground. Interception lightning protection can be provided for buildings, and in some situations for persons, by having an earthed conductor above the zone to be protected. Thus, the essential elements of an interception protection system are the air termination conductors to provide strike attachment points, the downconductors to convey the lightning current toward earth, and the earth electrodes to convey the lightning current into the general mass of the earth.

Because of their relatively high vulnerability to electric currents, persons are at risk of receiving a portion of the lightning current in situations that subject them to step potential and touch potential. They are also at risk of intercepting part of the lightning current flowing through water when swimming or wading.

Recommendations for personal safety in thunderstorms are based on the advice to recognize a high-risk situation and move from it to a lower-risk situation. Low-risk situations are those in which a direct strike to the person is prevented by a zone of protection provided by a nearby object, and there is no likelihood of the person being subjected to any portion of the lightning current flow by any of the mechanisms outline above. There are also engineering actions to reduce risk to persons inside buildings when using equipment with conducting connections to remote earth, in particular, the telephone.

Recommendations for the interception lightning protection of buildings are based on using existing building features as far as possible to provide the essential elements of a lightning protection system. These are the air termination conductors, the downconductors, and the earth electrodes. Buildings that do not have these features can be protected by appropriately positioned conductors and earth electrodes. It is fortunate that large, modern reinforced concrete buildings, or steel-framed buildings, with extensive metalwork on the roof are almost inherently protected against lightning damage, and will often only need bonding from roof metalwork to structural or reinforcing steel and protection against strikes to the sides to complete the interception protection system. Buildings with metal roofs, guttering, and downpipes may be close to being inherently protected against lightning. Buildings of mainly nonconducting materials are at some risk from lightning. It is likely that many houses and other buildings in cities are partly protected by nearby larger buildings and by overhead electric power distribution lines.

Protection of electrical equipment from damage by lightning is a field of engineering activity that has only been touched on briefly. In most situations, it is possible to provide adequate overvoltage protection for equipment to prevent lightning damage. However, in practice, it becomes an economic problem as to what expenditure is justified to prevent damage when the likelihood of lightning damage to any single item of equipment is low. In any given situation, engineering judgment has to be exercised to determine the extent of overvoltage protection that is justified.

REFERENCES

1. **Golde, R. H.**, Ed., *Lightning*, Academic Press, London, 1977.
2. **Uman, M.A.**, *The Lightning Discharge*, Academic Press, Orlando, FL, 1987.
3. **Golde, R. H.**, *Lightning Protection*, Arnold, London, 1973.
4. U.S. National Fire Protection Association, Lightning Protection Code, NFPA Publ. 78, Boston, 1969.
5. Lightning Protection, AS1768-1983, Standards Association of Australia, 1983.
6. British Standard Code of Practice for Protection of Structures against Lightning, BS 6651:1985, British Standards Institution, 1985.
7. Protection Contre la Foudre, Installations de Paratonerres, NF C17-100, Norme Française, Février, 1987.
8. **Berger K., Anderson, R. B., and Kröninger, H.**, Parameters of lightning flashes, *Electra*, 41, 23, 1975.
9. **Cianos, N. and Pierce, E. T.**, *A Ground Lightning Environment for Engineering Usage*, Stanford Research Institute Technical Report,1, August 1972.
10. **Anderson, R. B. and Eriksson, A. J.**, Lightning parameters for engineering applications, Electra, 69, 65, 1980.
11. **Standler, R. B.**, *Protection of Electronic Circuits from Overvoltages*, John Wiley & Sons, New York, 1989.
12. **Anderson, R. B. and Eriksson, A. J.**, A summary of lightning parameters for engineering applications, in Int. Conf. Large High Voltage Electric Systems, Paris, August 1980.
13. **Lee, R. H.**, Protection zone for buildings against lightning strokes using transmission line protection practice, *IEEE Trans. Ind. Appl.*, 14(6), 465, 1978.
14. **Darveniza, M. and Mackerras, D.**, Integrated lightning protection for large modern buildings, in *Proc. Inst. Eng. Austr. Electric Energy Conf. 1989*, Sydney, 1989, 131.

Chapter 10

LEGAL IMPLICATIONS OF LIGHTNING DAMAGE, INJURY, AND DEATH

Jon E. Krupnick, Kelley B. Gelb, and Jon D. Uman

TABLE OF CONTENTS

I. INTRODUCTION

Lightning has, since the beginning of time, been considered an uncontrollable force of nature, an act of God. Normally, this would mean there would be no liability for injuries, death, and property damage resulting from lightning. However, when an act of man acts concurrently with such an act of God, then liability may exist. This chapter will focus on the legal aspects of liability under tort law for lightning and telephone-related injuries.

Both state and federal courts have found that liability for such lightning injury, deaths, and damage exists under contract law (such as in the case of lightning insurance), statutory law (such as workmen's compensation laws), and under common law (such as the ever-increasing tort litigation). This chapter will focus primarily on the legal aspects of liability under tort law resulting from lightning strike and will attempt to bring to light some of the problems and hurdles to overcome in order to establish such liability.

It should be noted, however, that the concepts presented herein are those which are held in general, and although the American legal system is consistently striving toward national uniformity, every jurisdiction, whether it be local, state, or federal, varies in its common and statutory laws.

II. TORT LIABILITY

When, as the result of lightning, someone suffers some sort of injury or damage and that person is not protected by statute, such as in the case where one contracted with another to provide adequate lightning protection, then it is not immediately apparent that one may still seek relief under the law. After all, lightning has come to be known as an extraordinary, sudden, and unexpected manifestation of the forces of nature which man cannot resist. The reasonable interpretation of such an event would be that no one or no thing other than nature or perhaps God himself could possibly be held to blame.

Indeed, when the injury or damage is exclusively the result of a lightning strike, or any other direct, violent, and irresistible act of nature, it would be absurd to hold any human being liable. The law defines this "entire exclusion of human agency from the cause of injury or loss" as an "act of God", and it is, as such, an absolute defense to tort liability (1 Am. Jur. 675).

But, once someone with a responsibility to protect against such injury or damage has the reasonable opportunity to prevent such an outcome and does not take those steps toward prevention, the responsible party will be held liable if the actor's conduct was a "substantial factor" in causing the harm. It is generally held that if injury or damage results from the lightning strike and, concurrently, an act of negligence committed by a responsible person, such person cannot escape liability if the injury or damage would not have occurred except for the person's failure to exercise due care. (See, for example, *Bier v. New Philadelphia,* 11 Ohio St. 3d 134, 11 Ohio BR 430, 464 N.E. 2d 147 [1984]). In other words, once an intervening human agency contributes to cause the damage complained of, such damage cannot be said to have been caused by an act of God (*Cachick v. United States,* 161 F. Supp. 15 [D.C. Ill. 1958]).

In determining liability for lightning damage, then, the plaintiff must show that the defendant was concurrently negligent at the time of the lightning strike. In order to prove this concurrent negligence, the plaintiff must offer evidence that a party was responsible for the safety of those who were injured and that that responsible party did not exercise due care. Finally, if the responsible party breached its duty of care, the plaintiff must show that the injury or damage was proximately caused by the negligence. Several cases will serve to illustrate the intellectual process of the courts.

A. DUTY OF CARE

In *Davis v. Country Club, Inc.*, 53 Tenn. App. 130, 381 S.W. 2d 308 (Tenn. Ct. App. 1963), the plaintiff Davis took refuge in a wooden shelter on the country club golf course when a thunderstorm approached. The shelter, which had no lightning protection, was struck by lightning and Davis was injured. The court found first that since Davis was a member of the club and had therefore been invited onto the premises, the country club owed her the duty of exercising reasonable care to keep the premises in a reasonably safe and suitable condition, including the duty of removing or warning against a dangerous condition which it knew or, in the exercise of due care, should have known existed (*Id.* at 132, 381 S.W. 2d at 311).

But it was shown through evidence that the top of the wooden weather shelter was at a lower altitude than some of the surrounding rolling hills of the golf course. Expert testimony revealed that, all other things being equal, lightning would tend to strike a person, building, tree, or any other object in open country where the person, building, tree or object was higher than the surrounding ground (*Id.* at 311). After considering the evidence, the court found that the danger of the shelter being struck by lightning was so remote as to be beyond the requirement of due care and, therefore, the injuries and damages of the plaintiffs were not caused in whole or in part by any negligence of the defendants. Bare possibility is not sufficient (*Id.* at 311). The court went on to quote from the Supreme Court case of *Brady v. Southern R. Co.*, 320 U.S. 476 (1943), that events too remote to require reasonable provision need not be anticipated.

In *Brady v. United States*, No. 80-4156 (9th Cir. Dec. 30, 1981) (unpublished), the court found that although the National Park Service may not have been under the obligation to protect from lightning a certain hiking trail that led up the backside of a granite outcropping which apparently attracted lightning, the Park Service may, nonetheless, have been found negligent and therefore liable for the death of the plaintiff's decedent. who was struck and killed by lightning on the granite outcropping, because the Park Service made no attempt to warn visitors of the danger. *Tom on Torts*, 25 ATLA L. Rep. 241, 249, tells us it is basic negligence law that where the foreseeable harm is great, conduct threatening it may be held negligent, even though the statistical chance of its occurrence is very slight indeed. In other words, a slight chance of great harm can be condemned as an unreasonable risk, especially where the burden of adequate precautions (e.g., giving warnings) is relatively slight.

B. FORESEEABILITY

So we see that many courts look to the degree to which an event is foreseeable in determining the amount of action that is required of the defendant. The country club in *Davis,* although choosing not to protect the shelter from lightning nor to warn of the possible danger, was still found to have exercised enough care because the possibility that the shelter would be struck was too remote. But as *Brady* indicates, if the foreseeable harm were great, the defendant may have the responsibility to at least warn of the danger. In *Johnson v. Kosmos Portland Cement Co.*, 64 F.2d 193 (6th Cir. 1933), the Circuit Court explained the ways in which an event need be foreseeable in order to require action. In that case, the defendant company was the owner of a barge used to transport oil. After the oil had been unloaded, the hold where the oil had been stored was not properly cleaned out and gases generated from the remaining oil subsequently accumulated. When the barge was struck by lightning, the gases exploded and the plaintiffs' decedents were killed.

The court held that the fact that injury is the natural consequence of negligence is not enough; it must also be its foreseeable consequence. There is no actionable liability for an alleged negligent act unless injury resulting therefrom could reasonably have been foreseen in the light of attending circumstances (*Johnson* at 195). The court determined that the danger in permitting explosive gases to remain in the barge was obvious and that the defendant should have foreseen the consequences. The court went on to state that one need not foresee the particular way in which damage may result from his actions in order to be found negligent:

> We think the true rule to be that when the thing done produces immediate danger of injury, and is a substantial factor in bringing it about, it is not necessary that the author of it should have in mind the *particular means* by which the potential force he has created might vitalize into injury. (emphasis added) (*Id.* at 196).

Additionally, the court held that reasonable expectation of injurious consequences is not to be determined by the fact that no similar injurious result has been known to follow a like wrongful act under identical attending circumstances (*Id.* at 196). Simply because injury or damage has not resulted in the past does not mean it will not foreseeably occur in the future.

Courts in other jurisdictions, however, may not feel it necessary to consider foreseeability of injury as a factor to weigh in determining negligence. In *Bier v. New Philadelphia,* 11 Ohio St. 3d 134, 464 N.E. 2d 147 (Ohio 1984), the Supreme Court of Ohio indicated that there may be situations in which the defendant is held liable even though he may not have anticipated the damage resulting from the combination of the lightning and his own negligence. In this case, the Bier family had rented a metal-roofed picnic shelter from the city's park and recreation board. As a thunderstorm approached, the family began to pack up their picnic supplies. Before they were able to leave, however, lightning struck the shelter and the family was injured.

The court held that if the negligence of the defendants, namely, the failure to install a lightning protection system on the metal-roofed shelter, concurs with the other cause of injury, in point of time and place, or otherwise so directly contributes to the plaintiff's damage that it is reasonably certain that the other cause alone would not have sufficed to produce it, the defendant is liable notwithstanding he may not anticipate the interference of the superior force which, concurring with his own negligence, produced the damage.

C. NEGLIGENTLY INSTALLING EQUIPMENT

Once one assumes the responsibility to protect a house or other building from lightning and the building is thereafter damaged or destroyed, that responsible person may be held liable if the plaintiff can produce enough evidence to show that the responsible person was negligent in installing such equipment. In *White v. Schoebelen,* 91 N.H. 273, 18 A.2d 185 (1941), the court's ruling that the evidence showed that the "ground" was not "down to permanent moisture as required by state standards" was enough to affirm the judgment for the plaintiff property owner against the defendant lightning rod manufacturer, seller, and installer when lightning struck and set fire to the property.

Courts have held that although lightning rod companies contract with their customers to install such equipment and protect property, defendant installers may be held liable in tort because, as held in *Holmes v. Schnoebelen,* 87 N.H. 272, 178 A. 258 (1935), having undertaken to protect the building from lightning and, by necessary implication, the property of those who occupy it, the obligation arises not from the contract but from that action undertaken. This way, those who are not party or privy to the contract, but are nonetheless injured by the negligent installation of lightning protection systems, may recover under the law.

D. TELEPHONE CASES

Many of the injuries, deaths, and damages from lightning occur when lightning travels over telephone lines and enters the house or building that the lines enter. Most of the injuries and deaths result when someone is actually speaking on the phone when the lightning strikes. A great deal of damage is done as well when the lightning strike sets fire to that building into which the lines run; for example, when, through telephone company negligence, the lines are not properly grounded. The amount of care that the courts require of the telephone company to foresee and prevent such harm will largely determine the company's liability. When courts impose a higher standard of care upon the telephone company, the plaintiff finds it easier to show that the company was negligent. Defendant telephone companies much prefer the jurisdictions that hold the company to a lower standard of care, since the companies will have to exert less effort to satisfy their duty of care and the plaintiff will have to produce more evidence against the defendant in order to prevail. It is useful to explore the ways in which the standards of care vary from jurisdiction to jurisdiction.

The plaintiff's favorite scenario is that in which the telephone company is held to be an insurer of its product and, consequently, of the plaintiff against all injuries or damage. This would require the plaintiff only to show that the injury or damage was caused by or through the telephone equipment and not that the company was negligent in any way. It is generally held, however, that a telephone company, absent some sort of agreement to the contrary, is not an insurer against injury (*Chesapeake & Potamac Telephone Co. of Baltimore City v. Noblette*, 175 Md. 87, 199 A. 832 [Md. 1938]). Thus, in order to recover against a telephone company, the plaintiff must show that the defendant was negligent in not meeting the standard of care required by the court.

The court in *McDowell v. Southwestern Bell,* 546 S.W. 2d 160 (Mo. Ct. App. 1976), held that the defendant is required to use the highest degree of care practical in making safe the use of its phones (*Id.* at 166, quoting *Warren v. Missouri & Kansas Telephone Co.*, 196 Mo. App. 549, 196 S.W. 1030, 1031[1917]). In that case, the plaintiff brought an action against a telephone company to recover damages for injuries allegedly sustained by severe acoustical trauma. The plaintiff was talking on the telephone when he felt as if he had been "slapped" in the head, the alleged result of lightning traveling along the telephone lines to the telephone receiver. The court, in mandating that the telephone company use the highest degree of care, held that the telephone company has a duty to use known devices and methods to prevent the passage of dangerous amounts of sound (*Id.* at 165). In order for the plaintiff to show that the defendant breached its duty and was negligent under this standard of care, the plaintiff need only show that he was exposed to excessive noise or sound when using the telephone (*Id.* at 165).

In reaching its decision, the court cited other Missouri cases in which a person received an electrical shock while using the telephone and where the courts applied the same highest standard of care. The court reasoned that the duty to protect against excessive noise is the same as the duty to protect against electrical shocks.

The clear majority of courts, however, hold the telephone company to a less stringent standard of care. They require only that the telephone company exercise ordinary and reasonable care in maintaining its phone lines. One example is *Green v. Insurance Company of North America*, 275 So.2d 425 (La. Ct. App. 1973), cert. denied, 277 So.2d 672 (La. 1973), where the plaintiff brought suit for damages resulting from personal injuries she sustained while on the phone when lightning struck the telephone service line leading into her house. The court held that the telephone company must use reasonable and ordinary care under the circumstances to protect from injury (*Id.* at 428).

What, then, is considered "ordinary and reasonable care"? Many courts agree that if the harm is foreseeable, the telephone company must actually install protective devices. In *Griffith v. New England Tel. & Tel. Co.,* 73 Vt. 441, 48 A. 643 (1900), the telephone subscriber was sitting in his house underneath a wall-mounted phone when he was struck by a bolt of lightning and killed. The court held that if the telephone company:

> . . . had reasonable grounds to apprehend that lightning would be conducted over its wires to and into the house, and there do injury to persons or property, and there were known and approved devices for arresting or dividing such lightning so as to prevent injury therefrom to the house or persons therein, then it was the defendant's duty to exercise due care in selecting, placing and maintaining, in connection with its wires and instruments, such known approved appliances as were reasonably necessary to guard against accidents that might fairly be expected to occur from the lightning when conducted to and into the house over its telephone wires (*Id.* at 644).

Similarly, the court in *Southwestern Tel. & Tel. Co. v. Davis*, 156 S.W. 1146 (Tex. Civ. App. 1913), held that if the telephone company, in the exercise of due care, could foresee that lightning would travel into the house on the phone lines, then the company had a duty to install and maintain generally approved protective devices.

So we see that once the telephone company does install some sort of protection device, as is generally required, they may still be found liable if the plaintiff can show that the device was installed negligently (e.g., improperly grounded) or that the company was negligent in maintaining the lightning arrester in a reasonably safe condition and good working order at the time of the accident (*Whitehead v. General Telephone Co.*, 20 Ohio St. 2d 108, 254 N.E.2d 10 [1969]). This does not mean, however, that the law requires perfection beyond the limits of scientific knowledge and practicality as applied to an industry (*Green v. Insurance Company of North America*, supra). One need only employ the methods and appliances in general use by those engaged in a like business (*Rocap v. Bell Telephone Co.*, 230 Pa. 597, 79 A. 769 [1911]).

Since the telephone company is required only to protect its equipment and customers with standard protection devices in general use at the time, and that even with such devices correctly installed there remains some risk of danger involved while using a phone during an electrical storm, telephone subscribers are still subject to some danger. Given that most people are not aware of such a danger, it would seem that it would be logical to require the telephone companies to warn their subscribers of the danger. The courts, however, have not in fact required the telephone companies to warn the unwary public of this danger. The court in *Rocap* held that the failure of the telephone company to issue a warning against use during electrical storms was not sufficient evidence to establish negligence. The court also noted that no notice or warning has ever been placed by any telephone company on its phone warning of the danger of lightning.

III. CONCLUSION

As one can see by reference to all of the above, the outcome of cases seeking damages for injuries resulting from lightning strike are almost as difficult to predict as lightning itself. However, as a general rule, the negligence principles of foreseeability, ordinary care, and duty to warn can be used as guideposts to analyzing the cases.

Appendix 1

SPECIAL ASPECTS OF TELEPHONE-MEDIATED LIGHTNING INJURY — AN AUSTRALIAN PERSPECTIVE*

TABLE OF CONTENTS

* Reprinted from C. J. Andrews and M. Darveniza, *J. Trauma*, 29(5), 665, 1989. © Williams & Wilkins. With permission.

I. INTRODUCTION

Lightning has always been a possible hazard for people, property and electrical systems. Over many years, lightning protection has evolved to the stage where analytically-based engineering design can guarantee effective protection against most credible lightning flashes. This statement can be made with assurance for the lightning protection of buildings and of power system equipment. An element of uncertainty must however be accepted in the protection of telecommunication systems, because the modern solid-state equipment and its human users are more vulnerable to the effects of lightning. Of course, there will always be a possible hazard if no lightning protection is provided or if the protection installed is not fully effective.

There are about seven million telephones in Australia. Most are not provided with lightning protection, even in regions of moderate to high thunderstorm activity. The most likely reason for the lack of protection is that during the post-war period when the telephone system converted from overhead open-wires to buried cables, it was believed that the earth shielded the telephone conductors from lightning surges. This may be true for cables with metallic outer screens — but the Australian cables are mostly only surrounded by plastic sheaths. Further, and particularly in urban areas, the telephone network also includes sections of aerial cable.

Before 1980, records of injuries to telephone users possibly attributable to lightning were not available. In 1980, Telecom Australia started a new system for recording data of such injuries throughout Australia. In the period 1980 to 1985, 373 such cases were notified. No fatalities have been reported in Australia.

Also in 1980, Telecom Australia implemented a comprehensive policy of improving the lightning protection on the telephone system and of issuing warnings to users about the danger of using a telephone during a local thunderstorm.

The purpose of this appendix is to examine various aspects of telephone-mediated lightning injuries in Australia, particularly including medical aspects. The findings reported here are based on retrospective studies of the cases notified in Australia during the period 1980 to 1985.

II. MECHANISMS OF INJURY

There are several mechanisms by which the lightning current may enter a building.

A. DIRECT STRIKE

A direct strike to communication lines will obviously cause the impulse to impinge on a telephone user.

A direct strike to overhead power lines will similarly be transmitted into a building. From there it may be discharged to earth or by breakdown to communication lines.

B. INDUCTION

The electromagnetic field surrounding the lightning channel may induce current of considerable magnitude onto other conductors entering a building. Similarily currents travelling through conductors such as power lines may induce current onto adjacent conductors, possibly communication lines.

C. EARTH POTENTIAL RISE

In Australia, telephone equipment is not earthed at the subscribers termination, and is only earthed remotely at a telephone exchange. Any local earth potential rise will therefore set up a potential difference between local earth and the remotely earthed apparatus. A current may flow, due to this potential gradient, through any person in contact with the telephone apparatus.

TABLE 1
Australian Statistics of 328 Telephone-Related Lightning Incidents for the Period 1980–1985[1,3]

Parameter		Number	% of 328
State	Queensland	132	40
	New South Wales	73	22
	Western Australia	49	15
	Victoria	39	12
	Tasmania	22	7
	Northern Territory/South Australia	13	4
Area	Rural	149	45
	Non-rural	109	33
Thunderday level	< 30 pa	121	37
	30 pa	42	13
Soil resistivity	High	57	17
	Low	118	36
Telecom service	OH	175	
	UG	184	
Power service	OH	175	
	UG	19	
Telecom plant damage		113	34
Telecom protector fitted		30	9
Type of floor	Concrete	122	
	Non-concrete	112	
Discharge via	Electr. appliances	49	15
	Plumbing, etc.	42	13
	Floor	32	10
Shock	Electric	138	42
	Acoustic	67	20
	Both	80	24
Injury	Severe	—	10
	Minor	—	90

Note: Full information was not available for all the incidents.

III. AUSTRALIAN LIGHTNING INCIDENT STATISTICS

The data presented in the following are drawn from Telecom Australia sources[1-3] and from information provided to the authors during the execution of a current research project.[4]

The incidents, for which sufficient information are available, were analyzed on an Australia-wide basis,[1] and the results are given in Table 1. While the number of incidents may appear to be high for Australia's relatively small population (16 million) the rate is only about 0.000002% of all telephone calls. Even though such incidents are not rare events, their number is statistically small, and so their analysis may not produce meaningful correlations with such matters as, dependence on thunderday level, or soil resistivity, overhead versus underground Telecom cabling, rural versus non-rural area, etc. However, some findings are clear.

A.   A significant number of telephone-mediated lightning incidents (30 out of 328) have occurred even though lightning protectors were fitted to the telephone service. There are two explanations for this — either the protector was incorrectly fitted, or, and more probably, the protection was only partially effective because engineering practice current at the time of installation did not allow a bond to be made between the Telecom protector earth and the building's power earth. This isolation of the two "earths" can allow a potential difference between them if a surge current is injected into one (the engineering codes of practice now allow, and indeed recommend, that the two "earths" be bonded together).

B.   Nearly all telephone users involved in a lightning incident experience a shock; about 50% report perceived electrical shocks only, about 25% predominantly acoustic shocks, and the remainder experience a mixture of both. Acoustic shock may be caused by a sound pressure wave or by an electrical discharge to the ear. Many of the people who experience an electrical shock are "thrown physically", presumably by violent muscular reactions, and about 10% report being "knocked unconscious" for a short period of time. Somewhat surprisingly, only a small percentage (10%) report their injuries to be sufficiently severe to require medical attention.

C.   Only about 1 in 3 of the incidents were associated with damage to the Telecom plant (the telephone and/or nearby cable). This is not surprising as the majority of the reported injuries are minor. There appears to be correlation between the degree of injury and the extent of damage, and the most severe (for both) occur when the discharge path is mostly via conducting elements (such as 'earthed' electrical appliances or plumbing) rather than via wooden floors. In the case of the last, it is known that wood possesses a high impulse insulation strength[5] — at least 250 kV/m, even for wet wood. So, full-scale discharges are unlikely if the telephone user is separated from an "earth" by more than a meter of wood. This wood insulation does not however prevent a partial discharge of the local capacitor (of about 90 pF) formed between the telephone earpiece and the ear — the so-called capacitive spark, which because of its low energy is unlikely to cause significant physiological injury.

D.   The fact that no fatalities have been reported among the telephone users involved in the 328 lightning incidents calls for comment. Fatalities due to such incidents have been reported in other countries, e.g., in United States, one or two fatalities on average per year,[6,7] even though lightning protectors are widely used in that country. Why then have no fatalities been recorded in Australia? Certainly, some 10% of the injuries have been severe. A subjective assessment of some of the incidents and the medical reports leads to an inescapable conclusion — it is only a matter of luck that some of the more severe incidents did not lead to death.

IV. A RETROSPECTIVE SURVEY OF MEDICAL ASPECTS

A.   METHODOLOGY

A comprehensive questionnaire survey was undertaken of the 373 persons who notified Telecom Australia of a possible lightning incident mediated by telephone equipment between 1980 and 1985. Protocols for the issue of three questionnaires, and processing the responses, were developed which guaranteed confidentiality and consent from each person and which satisfied institutional and medical ethical requirements. The questionnaires were designed to obtain a medical history of the injuries and symptoms and other information considered to be relevant to each incident. Both specific and open-ended questions were asked. The responses were analysed by the research team, and were then evaluated medically (C.J.A.).

Table 2 lists the responses to the three questionnaires. Questionnaire 2 (Q2) was sent to non-respondents to the initial Questionnaire 1 (Q1), asked a substantially reduced set of questions, and was intended to elicit more responses. When a reply to Q2 was then received, Questionnaire 3 (Q3) was sent seeking to amplify the reduced information sought in Q2.

It should be noted that the type of questions used in the later Q3 were influenced by the information already gained from the original Q1, and so was more specific rather than open-

TABLE 2
Questionnaire Responses

Questionnaire	Sent	Received	Usable
1	335[1]	65	64
2	270	48	44
3	48[2]	24	24

[1] Because of incomplete addresses, questionnaires were not sent to 38 people involved in reported incidents.
[2] Sent only to questionnaire 2 respondents.

ended. A request was made to all respondents to consent to the release of medical records associated with the reported injuries and symptoms. One significant pattern of injury seemed to be related to the auditory apparatus, and so a number of respondents in southeast Queensland were invited to take audiometry tests.

B. RESULTS FROM QUESTIONNAIRE RESPONSES

The usable responses numbered 132 out of a possible total of 335, thus the information provided is the most comprehensive collection reported for a particular kind of lightning incident. It is possible however that the people who responded may not be fully representative of all involved in such incidents. Even so, the size of the response is sufficient to justify detailed analysis using standard statistical techniques and a method of cluster analysis.[8] Full details of the analyses are available from the authors. Here, we present a summary of the results based on an assessment of the combined information provided in the responses to the three questionnaires.

C. FREQUENCY ANALYSIS

Most of the responses were from adults (90%); about two-thirds were female; about two-thirds were from residences located in country postcode areas.

There is no clear pattern to the location of the telephone users at the instant of the lightning incident. Most were either standing or sitting, on a variety of floor types, and were touching a variety of household objects. Nearly all had the telephone touching an ear; about two-thirds were wearing shoes at the time. The data on various other aspects of the incidents are presented in Table 3.

The pattern of results for the questionnaire respondents in Table 3 does not appear to be substantially different from comparable results from Telecom Australia in Table 1 (for all incidents in Australia). This is an important matter for the purposes of this paper, because it suggests that the particular symptoms described by the respondents are representative of all the people involved in incidents and reporting to Telecom Australia.

The frequency analysis of symptoms in Table 4 are divided into two groups — immediate (short-term) effects, and longer term effects lasting for more than 24 h. It is of interest (and a surprise to the authors) to note that no medical aid was sought by about 60% of the people involved in the telephone mediated lightning incidents. Of the remainder, about 1/3 sought aid from more than one source (general practitioner or hospital) and about 1/5 were also treated by a specialist or a therapist.

D. CLUSTER ANALYSIS

Cluster Analysis is a numerical technique which aims to identify groups of injured people which most nearly resemble one another in terms of the constellation of symptoms they possess in common. The cluster analyses of the results were carried out and the resulting groupings

TABLE 3
Observational Statistics from Respondents

Variable	Numbers[1]	%
Loud noise heard in phone	35/108	32
Electric shock felt	38/108	35
Sparks from phone	22/108	20
Telephone damaged	26/108	24
Other equipment damaged	8/108	7.4
Person physically thrown	43/108	40
Subjective[2] extent of injuries		
Major	13/108	12
Minor	90/108	83
Nil	2/108	1.9
Subjective[2] duration of injury		
<24 hr	28/44	64
>24 hr	15/44	34
>3 months	2/44	4.5

[1] x/y indicates the number x who responded with a "yes" to a question about the particular variable; y is the number of responses to the particular question.

[2] In the view of the respondent or of another lay person.

TABLE 4
Symptom Frequency (Major Symptoms Only) Reported by Q1(64) and Q2/3(44/24) Respondents, Separated into Short-Term Effects (≤24h), and Long-Term Effects (>24h), with the Latter Subdivided into Three Groups
(S — 24h to 1w; M — 1w to 3m; L — >3m)[1]

Symptom	Short Term (≤24h) Number		Long Term (>24h) Number				
	Q1 (64)	Q2/3 (44/24)	Q1 (64)	Q2/3 (44/24)	S	M	L
Nil	4	0	20	8	—	—	—
Neurological System							
i) General							
Loss of Consciousness	10	5	—	—	—	—	—
Fitting	1	1	—	—	—	—	—
Headache	12	10	15	5	9	2	9
Memory loss	3	2	6	2	1	2	5
Confusion	5	7	—	—	—	—	—
Sleep Disturbance	—	—	9	4	6	1	4
Voice Abnormality	3	3	5	0	3	1	0
ii) Special Senses							
Otic							
Deafness							
ipsi	8	3	6	4			
both/unloc	4	6	5	3			
contra	1	0	0	0	5	5	11
loss discr	0	0	0	3			
Tinnitus							
ipsi	7	7	12	6			
both	0	9	5	2	11	7	12
unloc	0	1	5	1			
TMR/Bleeding	0	0	3	2			

TABLE 4 (continued)
Symptom Frequency (Major Symptoms Only) Reported by Q1(64) and Q2/3(44/24) Respondents, Separated into Short-Term Effects (≤24h), and Long-Term Effects (>24h), with the Latter Subdivided into Three Groups (S — 24h to 1w; M — 1w to 3m; L — >3m)[1]

Symptom	Short Term (≤24h) Number		Long Term (>24h) Number				
	Q1 (64)	Q2/3 (44/24)	Q1 (64)	Q2/3 (44/24)	S	M	L
Ocular							
Blurred vision	3	0	2	2 ⎫			
Pair	1	1	—	— ⎬	2	1	1
Other	2	1	3	0 ⎭			
iii) Motor/Sensory							
Weakness							
–Cranial N Region							
ipsi	2	0	1	6 ⎫			
unloc	0	0	1	0 ⎪			
–Spinal N Region				⎬	3	5	10
ipsi	8	5	6	4 ⎪			
unloc	1	0	0	0 ⎪			
–General/Unloc	11	6	0	0 ⎭			
Paraesthesiae							
–Cranial N Region							
ipsi	10	5	5	9 ⎫			
unloc	0	0	1	0 ⎪			
–Spinal N Region				⎬	9	5	9
ipsi	12	6	4	4 ⎪			
–General	5	4	0	0 ⎭			
Pain							
–Cranial N Region							
ipsi	16	4	10	12 ⎫			
both/unloc	8	1	4	0 ⎪	14	10	15
–Periph N Region				⎬			
ipsi	12	6	9	7 ⎪			
contra	0	0	1	0 ⎪			
gen	5	4	0	0 ⎭			
iv) Postural Control							
(Giddiness, Dizziness,etc)	13	14	13	8	8	11	12
v) Psychiatric							
"Shock"	19	15	2	0 ⎫			
Anxiety/Phobia	11	15	3	0 ⎬	5	1	7
Depressive Symptoms	0	0	7	3 ⎪			
Multiple/Other	0	0	1	1 ⎭			
CARDIORESPIRATORY SYSTEM							
Palpitations	11	6	1	1	1	1	0
Breathing impairment	6	2	0	0	0	0	0
INTEGUMENT							
Traumatic njury	7	0	3	0	3	0	0
Burns	6	7	0	0	-	-	-

[1] Duration, SML, of injury is summed over Q2/Q3 and Q1. The summation does not always equal the number of reported symptoms, since some respondents gave incomplete responses, or multiple responses with only one timescale indicated.

expressed in the form of a dendrogram.[8] The results are shown in the dendrograms for Q1 (Figure 1) and Q3 (Figure 2) responses and the data of significance for the three identified clusters are presented in Table 5.

E. CORRELATION ANALYSIS

Program SPSS (a standard statistical analysis package) was used to test for correlations between each of the symptoms and each of the observational variables elicited with the questionnaires. About 900 correlations were attempted for Q1 data, and 98 showed significance at the 5% level —one would expect 55 chance correlations at the 5% level. The numbers for Q3 are 660, 39 and 33. Thus, the correlations identified at the 5% level can only be assessed as having marginally more correlation than pure chance. The "most consistent" correlations were:

> Long term injuries with position of phone
> Many symptoms with position of phone
> Many symptoms with seeking more than one source of medical aid

F. MEDICAL REPORTS

In general, the 22 reports from medical advisers confirmed the history and information given by the patients in their responses. The authors believe that this provides verification of the validity of the questionnaire method used in this project.

The noteworthy differences were (1) two reports of ruptured tympannic membrane were not reported by the patients, (2) some indications of hypertension and tachycardia, and (3) two cases of audiometric loss.

The medical advisers' reports also exhibited differences in management and approach to the patients with lightning injuries. It was evident that most of the medical advisers involved had little clinical experience with such patients, a failing which the findings from this project should help to redress.

G. OTOLOGICAL EXAMINATIONS

All respondents in southeast Queensland, whether reporting ear problems or not, were invited to attend for audiometric examination: eight did. Rinne and Weber tests were performed and no gross abnormality in any patient was observed. Otoscopy and formal audiometry revealed no abnormalities attributable to lightning injury.

V. DISCUSSION OF MEDICAL ASPECTS

It is evident that the degree of injury suffered by a lightning strike victim must depend on the magnitude and the path of the impulse current causing the insult. A direct lightning strike exposes the victim to the full severity of the stroke current — the range of reported values is 3 to over 100 kA (average 30 kA). If the bulk of the stroke current passes through the body, the insult is catastrophic.

In contrast, the telephone-mediated incident is necessarily some distance from the point where the lightning strikes the ground. Thus only a fraction of the stroke current impinges on the victim — the fraction will be small if the distance to the strike point is more than 100 m. Even so, victims may be subjected to surge currents as high as 3 to 5 kA. But the target point is always the ear, a sensitive organ in itself, and located near other sensitive organs, eye and brain. The exit (or entry point) depends on which part of the victim's body is closest to an "earth" point. It may be the feet on a floor, or an arm, hand or back touching an earthed object (sink, refrigerator, etc.). Clearly, the current path always involves the head, the neck and the upper torso close to the cardiac and pulmonary systems. Thus, the path exposes critical parts of the human body to injury, even though the current magnitudes may be relatively small.

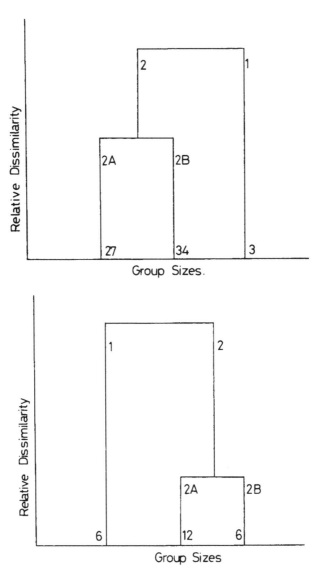

FIGURES 1 and 2. Dendrograms showing results of cluster analyses, and lightning flash syndromes, for Q1 and Q3 respectively, the most comprehensive questionnaires.

The authors have recently reviewed the medical aspects of direct strike lightning injuries (see Reference 9, which has an extensive list of references). Here, we compare the lightning injuries sustained while using a telephone with direct strike injuries.

The first and most obvious difference is the matter of mortality. As far as the authors know, no one in Australia has been killed by lightning while using a telephone, whereas fatalities are not uncommon for direct lightning strikes in the field.[6,7,9-11] The difference is clearly explainable by the relative magnitude of the surge currents involved in the two cases. For the same reason, the proportion of victims with serious injury is less for telephone mediated lightning incidents than for direct strikes. The respective percentages for loss of consciousness are about 15 and 60%. Cardiac arrest is quite common (20%) for direct strike victims, whereas none of the telephone users reported such an injury. Some of the telephone users reported less severe cardiopulmonary symptoms (palpitations and breathing impairment), and as expected these and other related symptoms are far more frequent for direct strike victims.

TABLE 5
Cluster Analysis of Q1(64)/Q3(24) Respondents (Summary Form[1] of Major Distinguishing Features)

Symptom or Variable	Cluster 2 61/8				Cluster 1	3/6
	2A	(27/12)	2B	(34/6)		
Variables						
Wearing shoes	+		+++		++++	
Damage to phone	o		+		++++	
Flooring	carpet=vinyl=concrete		carpet>vinyl>concrete		carpet++	
Victim's contact	metal		metal & wood		wood	
Victim thrown	+		++		++++	
Saw doctors	o		+		++++	
Short-term (<24-hr) symptoms						
Nil	++		o		o	
Neurological system						
Headache	+		++		+++	
Confusion	o		++		+++	
Voice abnormality	o		+		++	
Loss of consciousness	o		++		+++	
Tinnitus	++		++++		++	
Deafness	+		++		+	
Eye disorders	+		++		+	
Paraesthesiae	+		++		++	
Weakness	+		++		++	
Pain	+		++		++	
Postural control loss	+		++		++	
Shock	++		++		++++	
Psychiatric upset	+		++		+++	
Other symptoms						
Burns	+		++		o	
Breathing disorder	+		+		++++	
Trauma	o		+++		++	
Long-term (>24-hr) symptoms						
Nil	++++		o		o	
Neurological systems						
Sleep disorder	o		+	S	++++	SML
Headache	+	S	-	M	-	L
Voice abnormality	o		o		++++	L
Memory loss	o		+	ML	++	ML
Deafness	o		++	L	+++	SM
Tinnitus	-		+++	L	+++	M
Ocular disorder	o		o	S	++++	SML
Weakness	o		+++	SML	+++	ML
Paraesthesiae	o		+	SML	+++	L
Pain	+	S	++	M	++++	ML
Loss of postural control	o		+	SML	+++	ML
Emotional disorder	o		+	SL	++++	ML

TABLE 5 (continued)
Cluster Analysis of Q1(64)/Q3(24) Respondents (Summary Form[1] of Major Distinguishing Features)

Cluster size	40%	50%	10%
Cluster injuries	Minor Widespread	Moderate Short-term, widespread, longer-term otic/cns	Severe short-term emotional, longer-term widespread
Injury duration	<24 hr	24 hr-3 mo	>3 mo

[1] This table is presented in summary qualitative form using a five-point scale to indicate relative frequency within each cluster.

The relative magnitude of surge current is also the explanation of the differing extent of burns and other trauma experienced by the victims. A high percentage of direct strike victims (~40 to 60%) experienced such injuries, whereas only about 10% of the telephone users did. The pattern of significant difference between the two modes of lightning injury begins to change however when comparisons are made of specific symptoms related to the ears, the eyes and to the neurological system. For each mode, only about 10% of the victims experienced tinnitus, deafness or ruptured tympanic membrane. It would seem that the ameliorating effect of relatively small surge currents to the telephone user is compensated by the aggravating effect of specific target point (the spark between the telephone earpiece and the ear). It is very significant to any persisting symptoms and signs such injuries are strongly local and ipsilateral and this points to peripheral rather than central neurological injuries. This distinction is one of the major findings of this project.

Likewise, only a few percent of the victims from each mode of lightning injury experienced ocular symptoms. Visual loss, for varying durations, is the most common symptom, and for direct strike victims, there are some cases of physiological damage to the eye(s) especially long-term effects, like cataracts. The authors are pursuing this funding.

The same pattern of similarity seems to hold for certain specific neurological symptoms, namely paraesthesiae (including "numbness", "pins and needles", "burning sensations"), and weakness in various parts of the body. About 20% of the victims experience paraesthesiae in the ipsilateral head of neck, and the rate is much lower for other parts of the body.

It is much more difficult to make comparisons about the psychiatric effects experienced by the victims (anxiety, "shock", phobia, depression, etc. believed to be attributable to the lightning incident). Victims of both modes of lightning injury experience these forms of psychiatric disturbance. In both, their occurrence is quite common, and this is understandable. Fortunately, less than 10% experience long-term disturbances of a serious nature. Two main groups are noted; firstly, those who exhibit anxiety with some features of emotional lability, some with phobic aspects and many reporting "shock" (in the lay sense). Secondly, there are those reporting depression, changes in body image and regressive personality changes, often in the long term.

In contrast to direct lightning strike incidents, three distinct syndromes can be identified for the telephone-mediated lightning incidents. This identification is made from the cluster analysis. The first group is that of mimimal injury of short term duration; the second is of moderate injury of short to medium term duration, and the third is of severe injury with a tendency to long-term consequences. About 10% of the victims are in this severely injured category. It would seem that the degree of injury is related to the magnitude of the surge current imposed on the telephone user. It is usually impossible to determine the peak current retrospectively. But in those instances where this has been possible (the arc effects of impulse currents increase with peak current, and provide some quantitative measure), severe injury can be related to relatively large currents (3 to 5 kA) delivered to the ear of the victim.

VI. CONCLUSIONS AND PRELIMINARY TREATMENT RECOMMENDATIONS

This appendix has documented a major study of the degree and duration of symptoms and signs experienced by people struck by lightning while using their telephone. This area has received scant attention in the past and because of the recent upsurge in reports of such strikes, will become a more common problem for the primary care practitioner particularly. In general, injuries sustained have been shown to be relatively minor and of short duration. However, a small percentage suffer long term, severe and continuing disability.

A general division of injuries into three "lightning flash syndromes" has been made and the characteristics of each group have been given. Injury reports are, in general, diffuse, and ascription of precise etiology is difficult. Strong evidence exists that injury is of a peripheral rather than central nature.

It is appropriate to consider the factors which should guide a practitioner in assessing and treating such an injury. It is planned that a more comprehensive guide should be produced at a later date and reported in the normal manner, and the following represent preliminary remarks.

For the purposes of this section it will be assumed that the patient has recovered from any period of unconsciousness and that cardiac arrest (so common with direct strike but not found in Australia with telephone-mediated strike as yet) has not occurred. (In that case, of course, standard resuscitative measures should be employed.)

It is appropriate then for a practitioner to consider the following factors.

1. Cardiac status of the patient. Electrocardiography will reveal the presence of any arrhythmiae, and the unlikely presence of any signficant cardiac damage. Follow up should be advised.
2. Neurological status. The presence of local weakness, paraesthesiae, or pain will require careful examination to elucidate a cause.
3. Special senses. Early assessment by ear, nose and throat surgeons should be undertaken, if there is the slightest doubt about the status of the tympanic membrane, or the status of the patient's hearing, or any disorder of balance thought to be occasioned by the strike. The presence of tinnitus will similarly require assessment. Ocular assessment is desirable. While the authors have no reference nor survey finding for severe ocular damage, the potential exists injury for ocular damage. Base line assessment and continued observation are therefore advisable.
4. Psychiatric matters. Owing to the presence in some patients of psychiatric symptomatology, close primary care support over a period of time is considered appropriate. If problems arise then referral may well be considered. Preventive psychiatric intervention may be desirable.
5. Burns. Burns from direct lightning strikes have been referred to. Their severity is likely to be less for telephone mediated incidents. Such burns are mostly superficial and should be managed accordingly.
6. Investigations. It is not possible to indicate mandatory or even advisable investigations to fit all cases. Judgement must therefore be exercised as to appropriate investigations. However, the following may be considered: ECG, chest X-ray, serum electrolytes, full blood count, cardiac isoenzymes, urinalysis, and coagulation studies. CT scan may rarely be indicated. Audiometry may be useful.

ACKNOWLEDGMENTS

The work reported here was supported by grants from the Australian Research Grants Scheme. The authors acknowledge gratefully the assistance of colleagues, Telecom Australia staff, and the contributions from the people and their medical advisers who responded to our inquiries.

REFERENCES

1. **Bassett, P.,** *Analysis of Lightning Incidents,* Att 3 of "Customer Protection Against Lightning Injury", Report of all States Conference, Telecom Australia, Melbourne, 16-17 Sept. 1985.
2. **Johnstone, B. R., Harding D. L., and Hocking, B.,** Telephone Related Lightning Injury, *The Med. Jnl. of Aust.,* Vol 144, June 1986, p. 706.
3. **Schmidtchen, P. J.,** *Analysis of Customer Lightning Incidents,* Att 4, as for 1.
4. **Darveniza, M.,** *Electrical & Medical Effects of Lightning on People Inside Buildings in Australia,* Aust Res Grants Scheme, Grant 595, Univ of Queensland, Brisbane, 1986 & 1988.
5. **Darveniza, M.,** *Electrical Properties of Wood and Line Design,* University of Queensland Press, Brisbane, 1980.
6. **Bernstein, T.,** Effects of Electricity and Lightning on Man & Animals, *J. for Sciences,* Vol. 18, 1973, p1.
7. **Uman, M. A,** *All About Lightning,* Dover, 1986.
8. **Clifford H., et al.,** *An Introduction to Numerical Classification,* Academic Press, New York, 1975.
9. **Andrews, C. J., Darveniza M., and Mackerras, D.,** A review of medical aspects of lightning injury, *Adv. Trauma,* 4, 1989.
10. **Prentice, S. A.,** *Lightning Fatalities in Australia,* Electr. Eng. Trans., Inst. Eng. Aust., Vol. EE8(2), 1972, p55.
11. **Cooper, M. A.,** *Lightning Injuries — Prognostic Signs for Death,* Ann. Emerg. Med., 9, 134, 1980.

Appendix 2

FURTHER IDENTIFICATION AND TREATMENT MODALITIES IN TELEPHONE-MEDIATED LIGHTNING STRIKE

C. J. Andrews and M. Darveniza

TABLE OF CONTENTS

I. INTRODUCTION

In the previous appendix, the authors reported the results of a retrospective study of people who had been subjected to lightning strike delivered via their telephone lines. At that stage, it was pointed out that this phenomenon had been very little studied and represented a significant source of morbidity in the Australian environment. Since the writing of that appendix, the results have been updated and extended, and the object of this appendix is to present the new extensions.

The dearth of literature on the subject was alluded to previously. Most writers regard the "telephone-mediated" circumstance as only being an extension of an "in-the-field" lightning strike. The injuries are therefore presented merely as a further mechanism of more general field lightning injuries. Little attention is paid to the circumstance in its own right, and it has already been stated that significant differences exist in both the magnitude of the insult and the method of delivery of the injuring agent.

In recent literature, Eriksson and Ornehult[1] report the results of post-mortem examinations of lightning victims in Sweden. They cite two cases where victims died when subject to a lightning surge while using the telephone. Notable in this report is the immediate localization of all manifestations of injury to the face, head, and neck. This is strikingly consonant with the findings of the present study and will be alluded to later. It is also consonant with the previous study.

Frayne and Gilligan[2] also report a case of a man struck while using the telephone, and again the localization of his symptoms were to the head and neck, with a marked bias to neurological disability. A significant finding of the previous study was that the injuries were locally mediated rather than centrally mediated, although some personality change was noted, indicating a certain global element of cerebral damage.

The previous study was conducted in a retrospective fashion and therefore suffered from certain deficiencies. Marked among these deficiencies was the need for subjects to recall their injuries after a substantial period, and hence a degree of selective recall and inaccurate recall existed in the reporting process. There was also a degree of biased sample selection, and these problems were alluded to. The current research extensions aimed to rectify some of these deficiencies.

II. AIM OF RESEARCH EXTENSIONS

Bearing in mind the deficiencies of the previous sampling method, it was decided to gain access as quickly as possible to *all* persons who had recently been subjected to such an injury immediately after the injury occurred. The aim was thus to provide recent sampling of the complete spectrum of injury. It was felt that less bias would be introduced into the sampling process in terms of the tendency for more severely injured people to respond to a retrospective study, and that less recall problem in the reporting process would be evidenced. Also, when those injured were examined immediately, a more objective view of the injuries could be obtained by an external observer.

During three lightning seasons from 1988 to 1990 in the immediate regional vicinity of the authors' institution, 18 people reported lightning injuries to Telecom Australia; 12 were examined and 10 provided data suitable for inclusion in this study.

An immediate comment is made on these numbers. First, the total number receiving injuries over three lightning seasons is markedly lower than that discussed in the previous paper (approximately 30/year). The reasons for this are twofold. It is felt that Telecom has been actively monitoring this problem for at least 10 years, and in that time, people in areas of maximum risk have been supplied with protection for their telephone apparatus. Therefore, the remaining population is a relatively low-risk population. Further, a substantial public education program was undertaken during that time and substantial publicity given to the authors' research. Public behavior with regard to telephone usage during thunderstorms has been substantially modified. For these reasons, it is reasonable to expect the incidence of telephone-mediate lightning injury to have decreased markedly.

III. METHODOLOGY

This research extension relied heavily on the cooperation of Telecom Australia, which was willingly and readily forthcoming. Telecom Australia and the research team were at pains to be sensitive to issues of confidentiality. The participants in this prospective study were therefore guaranteed that their access to the research team was entirely confidential to the team, and the result of any examination was not made available to Telecom Australia. The mechanism for recognizing individual injured patients therefore took this into account.

During the period of the study, every person who reported an injury to Telecom had their incident investigated by Telecom Australia. At the time of this investigation, they were given a letter and verbal encouragement to contact the research team. The letter invited them to contact the research team as soon as possible to arrange an interview and examination with regard to their injuries. Cooperation was earnestly sought, and verbal encouragement to do so was provided by the Telecom investigator. Whether or not a person subsequently made contact with the research team, however, was a matter of individual initiative, and the Telecom officers had no knowledge of the decision. Confidentiality was thus assured.

All respondents who made contact with the research team were visited and examined immediately by a medical member of the team (C.J.A.). They were asked to consent to a medical examination which included electrocardiography and audiometry. In each case, consent was given. The two excluded patients came to the authors' notice outside this mechanism and, for the sake of consistency, were excluded from the study.

The response to the invitation in this study was double that of the previous study, and although the numbers are small, they represent a consistent cross-section of the injured population.

The mechanism was, however, not without minor criticism, and the major disappointment was the delay occasioned in some cases by some respondents in returning the form and making contact with the research team after the visit of the Telecom investigator. This was remedied part way through the study by providing respondents the option of returning the form to the research team via the Telecom investigator, should they so desire. The sacrifice in confidentiality was not considered by the majority to be of any moment.

The analysis to which the data were subjected aimed at identifying a particular risk group within the injured population. Cluster analysis was used in the previous study, and three lightning strike syndromes were identified. Data were accumulated in two ways. First, on the examination visit, information regarding the circumstance of the strike (physical details) was collected, as were comprehensive medical details of the injuries sustained. Subsequent to that, with the respondent's consent, a copy of the Telecom report of technical matters surrounding the strike was obtained and used to supplement the physical details referred to above. As these were more comprehensive than the subject's own assessment of the physical circumstances, the Telecom report was relied on heavily for the physical details.

Cluster analysis was applied to the subjects based purely on the medical details of their examination. This initial clustering allowed the grouping of individuals into categories of severity of injury. The physical variables derived from the Telecom report were then added to the data. Statistical analysis was applied to them to see if there were significant differences in the physical surroundings of particular strikes, given that the severity-of-injury categories had already been fixed. It was thus hoped to identify particularly risky circumstances based on the severity of injury sustained during the strike.

A second analysis was conducted for comparison purposes in which clustering was applied to the whole data set, just as in the previous study, with all the physical data included in the clustering process. This was done as a check on data consistency and for a wider view of the significant factors participating in the cluster process. The results were then compared.

IV. RESULTS AND DISCUSSION

A. NUMBERS

A gratifying high response was obtained with this methodology — approximately 60% of total strikes.This is roughly double the response obtained in the retrospective survey, and was felt to be an adequate response. Comments have already been made regarding the absolute size of this sample.

B. PRESENTATION OF DATA

An examination was made of the data in raw form, and this is presented in Table 1, which has been ordered to reflect the groupings later derived from the cluster analysis. The absolute symptoms that were seen mirror those noted in the previous study. Symptomatology was divided, as before, into short-term and long-term categories. The natural breakpoint for this was approximately 1 week for short-term injuries vs. greater than 1 week for long-term symptoms. The breakpoints for the previous study were 1 d, 1 week, and longer. However, examination of the data for this study showed the former to be a more natural division.

It was quite noticeable that the number of both short- and long-term symptoms reported were smaller than in the retrospective study. This is regarded as confirmation of the bias by which individuals magnify over a period of time the symptomatology that they had experienced a long time previously. The current set of symptoms, as found in this study, would seem to be a more realistic indication of the symptomatology of the injury.

Short-term symptomatology centers around three or four major areas. First, there is a group of ear symptoms appearing in three respondents, where pain, tinnitus, and altered sensation were noted. Second, a group of burns were seen, although only in two subjects. Facial, neck, and arm pain, including alteration in sensation, were seen in three respondents; however, psychiatric symptoms, largely centering around anxiety, were seen in six subjects, often to a marked degree.

Cardiovascular findings were evidenced in only three respondents, and consisted of tachycardia, which may well have been a manifestation of an anxiety state. Other minor symptoms, the largest of which was generalized musculoskeletal pain in three cases, was also seen. The duration of these initial injuries ranged from 1 to 5 d, with the majority less than 3 d.

Long-term symptoms were seen in only three of the ten subjects. This represents a larger percentage of the total that found in the previous study, where approximately 10% were found to have significant ongoing symptoms. Two of these three indicated marked psychological disturbance and problems have continued to date. The remaining symptoms centered entirely around continuing musculoskeletal pain, particularly in the arm, face, and neck.

Thus, a first conclusion is that the major long-term sequelae of this sort of lightning strike are pain (particularly musculoskeletal) and psychological disturbance.

C. CLUSTER ANALYSIS

The first analysis divided the subjects cleanly into two groups. Subjects 6 and 10 were one distinct group, and the remaining subjects formed the other distinct group.

Examination of these subjects' (6 and 10) data indicates that they are, in fact, two of the three subjects who demonstrated long-term and continuing upset. Thus, a predictor for severity of injury would seem to be duration of symptoms. It is interesting that subject 9 was left out of this cluster by the clustering process. However, examination of this subject's data shows that his continuing symptoms were mild and that the other two subjects were, in fact, quite debilitated. Once again, the major continuing problem was psychological upset and pain. In the case of subject 9, psychological upset was not as prominent.

TABLE 1
Raw Symptom Summary

Parameter		1	2	3	4	5	7	8	9	6	10	Key
Short-Term Symptoms												
				(Not significant, $p < 0.05$)								
Loss of Conc.		A	N	N	N	A	A	A	Y	A	N	A = altered conc., Y = yes, N = no
Ear	Paresthesia	+									++	
	Pain		+								+++	
	Tinnitus	+	+									
Burns	Presence	Y			Y				Y			1 = arm, leg, chin; 2 = mouth; 3 = singed hair
	Site	3			1				2			
Arm	Paresthesia									++	++++	
	Pain									++	++++	
Facial swelling		+									++	
Nausea/pain abdomen			N						P	P		N = nausea, P = pain
Tachycardia								++	+		+	
Hemoptysis									+			
Muscular pain							1,3	1	2		3	1 = thorax, 2 = back, 3 = neck
Duration of initial symptoms		5	2	0	2	0	3	1	3	1	3	(Days)
Long-term Symptoms												
				(All significant, $p < 0.05$)								
Nil		Y	Y	Y	Y	Y	Y	Y				

TABLE 1 (continued)
Raw Symptom Summary

Parameter	Respondent										Key
	1	2	3	4	5	7	8	9	6	10	
Duration								C	C	C	Currently continuing
Psych. upset									+++	+	
Abdominal pain								+	+		
Arm Pain/Paresthesia									+	+++	
Arm Weakness										+++	
Headache									+		
Muscular pain								+		+++	
Examination:	In all cases, objectively normal										
Telcom "physical" data (supplemented by team data)	(* = significant, $p < 0.05$, analysis 1; + = significant, $p < 0.05$, analysis 2)										
Location	U	U	R	R	U	U	R	U	S	U	U = urban, S = suburban, R = rural,
Topography	F	H	F	U	F	F	H	F	H	U	U = undulating, H = hilly, F = flat
Distance to nearest hill		20		200					25		
Storm intensity	L	L	L	L	M	S	S	M	?	L	L = light, M = moderate, S = severe
Concurrent lighting	N	M	O	O	M	N	F	F	?	O	L = light, O = occas, M = mod, F = freq
Strike distance	400	N	N	N	N	200	N	250	25	N	N = not known; otherwise meters
Local storm history	M	M	L	?	L	M	M	L	M	M	L = light, M = moderate
Power system Feed	O	U	O	O	U	O	O	U	O	U	O = overhead
Power system Retic	O	U	O	U	U	O	O	U	U	U	U = underground
Damaged in strike	N	N	N	N	N	N	N	N	Y	N	* + } Y = yes
Appliances damaged	N	Y	N	N	N	N	N	N	N	Y	* + } N = no
Phone Feed	U	U	U	O	U	U	U	U	U	U	O = overhead
Phone Retic	U	U	U	O	U	U	U	U	U	U	U = underground

Variable											Key
Phone damage	1	3	0	1	1	0	0	4	0	3	Scale, 0—4
Building constr.	B	B	T	B	B	B	F	B	B	C	F = fibro, B = brick, C = concrete
High (H)/low (L) set	L	L	H	L	L	L	L	L	L	H	
Roof	M	T	M	?	T	M	M	M	T	•	M = metal, T = tile, • = not applicable
Building frame	M	T	T	T	T	T	M	M	T	?	? = unknown
Floor height	O	O	A	O	O	O	O	O	O	A	O/A = on/above ground
Floor material	C	C	T	C	C	T	C	C	T	C	T/C = timber/covered concrete
Body contact	O	O	O	G	O	P	P	P	P	G	G = good, P = poor, N = no earth
Shoes	N	N	N	Y	N	Y	N	Y	Y	Y	+
Handset thrown	Y	N	Y	Y	D	D	N	Y	N	Y	Y = yes, N = no, D = dropped
Service made faulty	Y	Y	N	Y	Y	N	N	Y	N	Y	
Sparks seen	N	N	N	Y	Y	N	N	Y	Y	N	
Self thrown	N	Y	N	N	N	N	N	Y	N	Y	+
Acoustic shock	3	3	0	0	0	2	1	0	0	0	Scale, 0—3

Each of the data items contributing to the cluster analysis were then examined for statistical significance between the two groups. All the variables representing long-term symptomatology were significantly different ($p < 0.05$) between the two groups. Further, the only variables in the short-term symptomatology that were significantly different between the groups were those representing arm pain and altered arm sensation. In this study, these particular variables could be used as discriminators for long-term injury and thus severity of injury. It was noticeable that none of the physical circumstances discriminated between the particular groups (initially based on the physical data collected by the author).

When the physical variables collected by Telecom Australia were added to the study, only two reached significance — those relating to associated power system damage with the given strike. Particularly, there was no significance to variables such as storm intensity, storm history, phone line construction, housing construction, or terrain. The fact that these variables did not reach significance may be a reflection of the small sample size. However, consistent significance with associated power system damage adds credence to the stated Telecom Australia view that entry into a dwelling via an associated power system strike is a highly important means of entry of the injuring impulse. Further comments on this matter will be made later.

The second analysis allowed the clustering to proceed on the basis of all variables, including Telecom physical data. The clustering in this process showed an almost identical division into two cluster classes. This time however, subjects 6, 9, and 10 were clustered into a group of greater severity than in the first analysis. In retrospect, it was noted that subject 9 only joined with the lightly injured group at a very late stage in the clustering process in the previous analysis, and so may be regarded as "a floater". Once again, the division on severity of injury is made on the basis of long-term symptomatology alone, and these are the only medical variables which reached statistical significance.

In the second case, the physical data of significance also included whether the victim was wearing shoes or not. This may well represent a chance association. However, the analysis shows that, statistically, severity of injury is *positively* associated with the wearing of shoes. This may represent a tendency to capacitive coupling to the impulse rather than direct conductive coupling. One author (M.D.) has previously drawn attention to the phenomenon of a "capacitive spark", as opposed to a "conductive spark".

The only other variable shown to be of significance in this second analysis was whether the victim was thrown by the impulse. This would seem to be a natural correlate of severity of injury, and could well indicate a degree of musculoskeletal trauma which could give rise to long-term musculoskeletal disability.

V. IMPRESSIONS FOR THERAPY

In this study, as in the previous study, injuries, particularly those of severe degree, are local to the passage of electric current and are not derived from a central causation for continuing symptomatology.

Subsequent to this study, the author has been called upon to treat a number of these victims, something which was specifically precluded in the previous research methodology. Having completed the study, it was felt by the first author that he was ethically able to undertake such treatment.

The major features of injury are psychological and musculoskeletal. And this finding of the study has been borne out as an impression of the presentation of these people clinically. Further clinical impressions are now described.

The pain with which the victims present is very local to the line of the strike. It is felt to have been neuritic in origin, i.e., derived from direct peripheral nerve cell damage. This is borne out by the clinical nature of the pain and by a plausible connection with the passage of electric current, i.e., the electric current specifically and selectively damages the sensory nerve terminals and peripheral sensory neural conducting pathways which are traversed by the current. This is further borne out by the success the first author has had in treating these injuries with carbemazepine and/or clonazepam. These are agents known to be of particular use in neuritic pain. A standard dose regimen has been used, gradually decreasing the dosage until the minimum to achieve control is found. Although the symptoms lasting greater than 1 week have been classified as long term, in fact they appear to improve gradually over 6 to 8 months, and the need for medication is finally removed.

Psychological factors are seen to be prominent when these people present, and it is a clinical impression of the first author that the majority of people with continuing problems have a more obsessional type of personality. This is not necessarily derived from the current data. It represents a clinical impression and is a plausible extension of the anxiety states seen in this study. The obsessional personality finds it difficult to cope with situations beyond immediate control. Issues of control of destiny and health are very strong in the obsessional. Many of the patients report frustration at having continuing problems they do not understand and that are foreign to their experience. In their perception, the loss of control is made worse because "no one else seems to understand" the syndrome either. They feel that the good health they had been totally in control of previously has now been independently snatched from them, and this created anxiety in itself, and particularly anxiety generated by being subject to the unknown. All this plausibly connects with psychological feelings of ongoing anxiety and mixed anxiety depression. The author has therefore found it useful to add a degree of tricyclic antidepressant medication (particularly clomipramine) to the above pain relief. The basis for doing this is to provide relief from the obsessional features of the psychological disturbance as well as to provide primary antidepressant action. Tricyclics also are known to be useful adjuncts to pain relief modalities. Thus, the regimen of antineuritic pain relief and antidepressant therapy has come close to being the author's standard.

VI. IMPLICATIONS FOR PROTECTION STRATEGIES

It was hoped that this study would indicate clearly particular groups of subjects who were at risk of injury due to their physical circumstances, and thus allow the authorities to concentrate on protecting such individuals. This has not turned out to be the case. The only positive association which could be drawn from the study was the association with power system strikes and the severity of cross-coupling between the power system and the telephone system. This is something that is not altogether unknown already. Perhaps the study can be regarded as providing positive reinforcement for the insistence on earth bonding between the telephone system and power supply system by Telecom as a matter of priority in service protection.

Particularly, no geographical or terrain feature, or feature of storm intensity has been found to be significant in this study, even though the number were small. The only formal parameter not measured has been earth resistivity; otherwise, the study is felt to have been comprehensive.

VII. CONCLUSIONS

This study has provided the first detailed prospective examination of people struck by lightning which was mediated via the public telephone system. It has had a gratifying high response and, in the current Australian climate, represents a comprehensive examination of the injuries. The broad findings of the previous retrospective study have been confirmed in that the majority of injuries seen, particularly those of severe degree, are local to the line of current and not mediated centrally. The best predictors of severity of injuries and their duration are the presence of musculoskeletal pain and the presence of symptoms lasting longer than possibly 3 d, and at least 1 week. The major physical parameter found to be of significance in predicting injury severity has been the presence of power system damage, and this provides a measure of reinforcement for the current policy of regarding earth bonding as a significant step in system protection. Impressions for treatment have also been given, particularly the recommendation that antineuritic pain relief and antidepressant therapy be used.

REFERENCES

1. **Eriksson, A. and Ornehult, L.,** Death by Lightning, *Am. J. Forens. Med. Pathol.,* 9(4), 295, 1988.
2. **Frayne, J. and Gilligan, B.,** Neurological Sequelae of Lightning Stroke, *Clin. Exp. Neurol.,* 24, 195, 1988.

Appendix 3

AN AUSTRALIAN REPORTING PROCEDURE AND STATISTICS

B. Hocking

The proper analysis of lightning-related telephone injury reports is important in directing and monitoring control procedures. The quality of the database will be directly influenced by the quality of the reporting systems and, to a lesser extent, by social factors such as media publicity or increased warnings to the user about lightning-related injuries.

Reports may be analyzed by absolute numbers, as shown below. In many situations, however, it is better to express them as a rate to allow for the extent of public exposure. The easiest obtainable unit of exposure is the number of telephone services in a country or area. In some countries, e.g., U.S. and Australia, nearly all homes and workplaces have a telephone; but in others, e.g., Russia, there are much fewer (World Telecommunications). Therefore, the possibility of an incident is greater in the former countries. This variation between and within countries needs to be taken into account when making comparisons, as shown below. A further estimate of exposure would be the number of telephone calls made in a year, although the introduction of FAX services will lessen the extent of human exposure while increasing the number of calls.

In Telecom Australia, data for 426 consecutive reports are available from January 1980 to December 1987, as shown in the accompanying figures and table. Table 1 shows the distribution of reports by year and state. Figure 1 shows the national figures for the 8 years expressed as a rate per million telephone services. The low rate in 1980 probably reflects underreporting at commencement of the database. The downward trend thereafter may possibly be due to the success of the control strategy.

Figure 2 shows the distribution of all reports by state expressed as a rate, using the mid-point 1984 number of services in each state to calculate the rate. The high rate in Queensland is compatible with high keraunic activity in that state. The high rate for Tasmania should be interpreted with caution because of the small number of reports (25).

Figure 3 shows the distribution of reports by month. The high numbers in December and January relate to the cyclone season in Queensland with high lightning activity.

Thus, analysis of data by time and space can provide useful data for understanding causes of the problem, directing preventive activities, and monitoring the efficiency of control procedures.

REFERENCE

World Telecommunications 1987-88 Fact Book, Telecommunications Industry Research, Barnham, U.K.

TABLE 1
Lightning Statistics

Year	Aust.	NSW	VIC	QLD	SA & NT	WA	TAS	Number of SERVICES ('000)
80	10	2	2	4	2	0	0	4743
81	94	10	8	51	3	10	12	5069
82	36	10	2	18	0	3	3	5357
83	65	20	10	27	2	6	0	5592
84	61	15	12	16	2	10	6	5851
85	70	13	18	26	5	5	3	6188
86	38	3	14	14	4	3	0	6501
87	52	6	15	23	0	7	1	6816
Totals	426	79	81	179	18	44	25	

Note: NSW, New South Wales; VIC, Victoria; QLD, Queensland; SA, South Australia; WA, Western Australia; TAS, Tasmania.

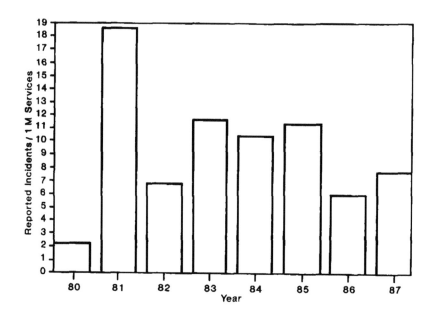

FIGURE 1. National annual rate per 1 M services.

189

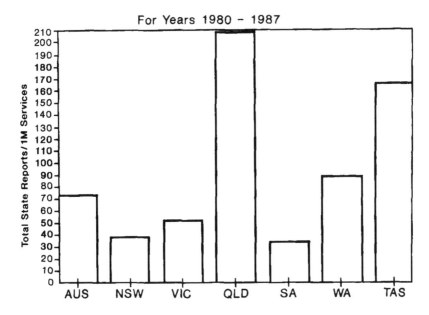

FIGURE 2. Reports by state per 1 M services for years 1980 to 1987.

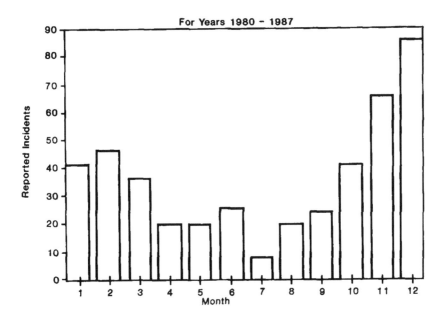

FIGURE 3. Monthly lightning report patterns for years 1980 to 1987.

INDEX

A

Acoustic energy, 17
Acoustic shock, 18
Acoustic wave, 17
Action integral, 17
"Act of God", 88, 91, 158
Aerosol particles, 11
Airplane wings, 17
Air termination network, 153–154
Alanine aminotransferase (ALAT), 111
ALAT, see Alanine aminotransferase
Aldolase, 109
Amnesia, 59, 88
Animals, 18, 31–32
Antennas, 18
Anterograde amnesia, 59
Antibiotics, 131, 134
Anxiety, 89–90
Arc discharge path, 29–31
ASAT, see Aspartate aminotransferase
Aspartate aminotransferase (ASAT), 109
Attachment process, 14, 146
Audible thunder, 16, 17

B

Bier v. New Philadelphia, 158, 160
Blast damage, 28
Blindness, 18, 59, 89
Brady v. Southern R. Co., 159
Brady v. United States, 159
Building features and protection from lightning, 154–155
Burns, 62–67, 101–108, 120, 122, see also specific types
  contact, 66, 67, 101, 104
  corneal, 60–61
  deep, 67
  entry-point, 104–108
  exit-point, 104–108
  feathering, 63, 67, 68
  flash, 67, 101
  follow-up for, 143
  full-thickness, 64, 101, 135
  linear, 65, 67, 68, 101–102
  partial-thickness, 135–136
  streaking, 62
  treatment of, 130, 134–136
  types of, 62
Bystander response, 118

C

Cachick v. United States, 158
Capacitance, 24, 35–36
Capacitors, 24, 32
Cardiac arrest, 4

Cardiopulmonary resuscitation, 118, 130, 134
Cardiorespiratory arrest, 82
Cardiovascular symptoms, 53–55, 80
  follow-up for, 142
  treatment of, 122–124, 127–128
Case studies, 50–53
Cataracts, 18
Central nervous system symptoms, 84–85, 94, 125–126
Charcot's paralysis, see Keraunoparalysis
Charge generation, 10
Charge transfers, 11, 17, 18
Chesapeake & Potomac Telephone Co. of Baltimore City vs. Noblette, 161
Cloud-to-air discharges, 12
Cloud charge dipole, 10–11
Cloud-to-cloud discharges, 12
Cloud discharges, 12
Cloud electric fields, 10
Cloud-to-ground (streaked or forked) lightning, 12, 13–16
Cloud types, 9–10
Cluster analysis, 167, 170, 180, 184
Cochleovestibular symptoms, see Otologic symptoms
Collectors, 25
Complement activation, 109
Conductivity of soil, 18
Conductors, 24, 25, 35–36, 146
Confusion, 60, 68, 88, 89
Consciousness loss, 88, 118, 120
Contact burns, 66, 67, 101, 104
Convection theories, 10–12
Corneal grafts, 131
Correlation analysis, 170
Corticosteroids, 131
Countershock, 80
CPK, see Creatinine phosphokinase
Creatinine phosphokinase, 11
"Crispy critter" myth, 3
Cross-sectional areas, 24
Current, 30, 32, 77
  direct, 80
  discharge, 147
  distribution of, 73
  effects of flow of, 27–32
  effects of on structures, 148–150
  electrical aspects of, 24
  ground, 82
  integral of, 17
  interception of, 147
  internal, 78
  lightning stroke as source of, 25–27
  magnetic field of, 32
  magnitude of, 24, 74
  maximum rate of change of, 17
  measurement of, 32
  mechanisms for production of, 147–148

Milton Keynes UK
Ingram Content Group UK Ltd.
UKHW052017071024
449327UK00027B/2313